C000217840

WHOSE BODY IS IT ANYWAY?

A Sociological Reflection upon Fitness and Wellbeing

Ian Wellard

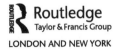
Routledge
Taylor & Francis Group

LONDON AND NEW YORK

First published 2019
by Routledge
2 Park Square, Milton Park, Abingdon, Oxon OX14 4RN

and by Routledge
711 Third Avenue, New York, NY 10017

Routledge is an imprint of the Taylor & Francis Group, an informa business

© 2019 Ian Wellard

British Library Cataloguing-in-Publication Data
A catalogue record for this book is available from the British Library

Library of Congress Cataloging-in-Publication Data
Names: Wellard, Ian, author.
Title: Whose body is it anyway? : a sociological reflection upon fitness and
    wellbeing / Ian Wellard.
Description: Abingdon, Oxon ; New York, NY : Routledge, 2019. |
    Includes bibliographical references.
Identifiers: LCCN 2018025983| ISBN 9781138959507 (hardback) |
    ISBN 9781138959514 (pbk.) | ISBN 9781315660608 (ebook)
Subjects: LCSH: Physical fitness—Social aspects. | Well-being—Social
    aspects. | Body image—Social aspects.
Classification: LCC GV342.27 .W45 2019 | DDC 613.7—dc23
LC record available at https://lccn.loc.gov/2018025983

ISBN: 978-1-138-95950-7 (hbk)
ISBN: 978-1-138-95951-4 (pbk)
ISBN: 978-1-315-66060-8 (ebk)

Typeset in Sabon
by Swales & Willis Ltd, Exeter, Devon, UK

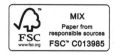
MIX
Paper from
responsible sources
FSC
www.fsc.org   FSC™ C013985
Printed in the United Kingdom
by Henry Ling Limited

WHOSE BODY IS IT ANYWAY?

There is a widespread interest in wellbeing, the healthy body and public health. However, there are also many simplistic and uncritical interpretations of what wellbeing or a healthy body should 'look like'. By focusing upon wellbeing through examples taken from fitness-related activities, which are often considered unproblematic routes to achieving wellbeing and greater public health, this book explores contemporary understandings of the body and the conflicting ways in which it is considered, in different contexts, times and spaces, either as the possession of the individual or that of society (or both).

Whose Body Is It Anyway? adopts an embodied approach, employing sociological theory along with examples drawn from empirical research collected through participation (by the author) in an intense period of physical training. The intention is to explore the embodied experiences of 'doing' an intensive period of physical activity and, subsequently, attempt to understand, in more depth, the range of personal, social, psychological and physical factors that undoubtedly contribute to engaging in such an activity.

The emerging story reveals much about the physical and emotional experience of a body being put through intensive exercise, not only in terms of contrasting forms of pleasure and pain, but also various socio-cultural 'issues' relating to relationships of power, trust and the role of 'expert' health advisor. Written in a clear and engaging style, the book provides an accessible introduction of more complex theoretical explanations which will appeal to academics and practitioners involved in broad aspects of sport, physical activity, health and wellbeing.

Ian Wellard is a sociologist of Sport and the Body. His main research interests relate to embodied practices, physical activity, gender and sport. Much of this research has been generated through ethnographic studies, which draw upon qualitative and reflexive approaches to the ways in which embodied identities are constructed and negotiated. His previous publications include *Researching Embodied Sport* (2015), *Sport, Fun and Enjoyment* (2013), *Sport, Masculinities and the Body* (2009) and *Rethinking Gender and Youth Sport* (2007), all published by Routledge.

CONTENTS

ILLUSTRATIONS

Figures

Tables

ACKNOWLEDGEMENTS

I would like to thank Routledge for their continued support. I know that what I like researching and writing about does not always follow the current trends, so I am grateful that they consider me worth the risk.

I would also like to thank those who have helped me in my thinking over the last couple of years. In particular, Lucy, James and the other James, who between them managed to bring CrossFit to my attention and help me find something to fill the gap left after having to give up tennis.

Lastly, I would like to thank John (again) for his patience and support and Toby whom we miss like mad.

1

INTRODUCTION

In this book, I explore how contemporary knowledge about the body shapes the way in which it can be experienced in different contexts, times and spaces as either the possession of the individual or the possession of society (or both). I examine these ideas through the central theme of sport and physical activity, which is an aspect of contemporary life that is often considered to be an automatic pathway to wellbeing. In this formulation of wellbeing, the notion of having a healthy body or a sporty body is often in direct contrast to an unhealthy or non-sporty body. This simplistic binary provides a useful mechanism to explore the contradictions and tensions that lie beneath the surface, allowing opportunities to assess the ways that the social body operates to 'look after' the individual while, it could be argued, at the same time imposing restrictions on how the body can operate at an individual level. However, a binary of sporting and non-sporting participation (those that do and those that do not want to), which is often cited in many public and academic spheres, does not allow for a more nuanced consideration of the conflicting ways in which knowledge is generated and subsequently interpreted by an individual. Within professional health circles the focus is invariably on those who are less active and, consequently, perceived as a problem. The proposed remedy is to provide measures to engage them in physical activity. In many cases, critical reflection is not made about what it is they should be doing or what, indeed, the experience of getting active actually means to someone who does not find the idea of being active appealing. Likewise, there is often an unquestioned assumption that what 'sporty' people are doing is always necessarily healthy.

Underlying all of these assumptions is knowledge about health, generated through formulations of science and medicine, which specifically focuses on biological prescriptions of what a healthy body should look like and how it should behave. In order to acknowledge the influence of sociological and historical elements within these bio-scientific understandings, I have drawn on the example of contemporary sport and fitness practices to reveal the competing factors that influence the way we view and make sense of our own bodies and those of others. Incorporation of an embodied approach allows the introduction of more complex theoretical explanations, which are crucial in our attempts to understand what shapes our perceptions of healthy activity and, ultimately, the extent to which we have a say in whose body it is anyway.

Although I acknowledge that the central focus of this book is ambitious, it is not my intention to provide an extensive genealogy of health and sport in the way that other sociologists and historians have previously attempted. As indicated above, my primary motive has been to 'raise questions', which are not necessarily new, but are, nevertheless, often overlooked or even ignored. Although there has been much written about knowledge structures relating to the body (Foucault 1978, Frank 1990, Shilling 1993), health and bioscience (Rose 2007) and sport (Hargreaves 1986), these are from what might be described as a broader post-structural standpoint (Howarth 2013). However, although they make my task easier in that they have provided a substantial theoretical foundation, my approach has been to incorporate a much more reflexive context, where personal embodied experiences that have influenced subjective interpretations of health, wellbeing and sporting participation ultimately generate further questions that I attempt to explore within this book.

My body as a mechanism to understand others

I have always found the body fascinating. Not that I am suggesting I am the only one who does, as I am sure many others do too. When I say that I find it fascinating, it is through a sociological lens where the academic training that I have had during my life has provided opportunities to explore in detail my broader interests in a social body that I was aware of from an early age. I can remember being interested in the ways that bodies moved, presented themselves and could actually 'be'. I was vaguely aware of how I was constantly performing with and through my body. This also appeared to be the case with others and I tried to understand a 'performing' body, often considered problematic, and which should be constantly negotiated or even hidden.

Without doubt I consider the early experiences of my body, along with an awareness of other bodies, having shaped the way that I have been able to develop a theoretical approach and formed subsequent explanations for it. These experiences have influenced my perceptions and the way that I choose to theorise. Although I seek to accommodate sociological thinking I am, nevertheless, influenced by a range of other, sometimes contradictory, explanations, which emerge from philosophy, physiology and history. At the same time, I do not feel the need to make futile attempts at claiming or making claims for objectivity. By detailing (and revealing) my subjective experience, I acknowledge that what I write within this book is a subjective account of my understanding and interpretation of the social body. However, much of the material that I draw on has been collected using traditional sociological methods and I adhere to many traditional forms of sociological data collection to lend support to my theorising. For instance, some of the material presented in this book has been drawn from ethnography, qualitative interviews, observations and research diaries. The important point here is that in this introduction I am trying to offer a glimpse into the ways in which I have been able to develop my train of thought. I am aware that many readers may not always agree with the arguments put forward but it is important to establish a context for these thoughts. Nevertheless, it is also important to note that I do not see my experiences and thoughts as entirely different to anyone else's. The very fact that we do 'have' a body that is formed physiologically in very similar ways, and that we are exposed to social structures and discourses that shape the way we are able to think and interpret the world, suggests to me that subjectivity and personal experience do not necessarily equate to purely subjective and meaningless (to others) ideas.

My initial fascination with the body generated many questions that I was constantly trying to unravel as a teenager. There appeared to be so many contradictions in terms in what I could do with my body and, similarly, what my friends could do with their bodies. Sometimes it seemed that we did have unlimited freedoms. We could choose to run as far as we wanted until we were too tired to run any further, we could stuff our faces with chocolate until we could eat no more.

Like everyone, there are undoubtedly many experiences that stand out in my personal history that have either changed my way of thinking or exposed me to different ways of 'seeing' the world. Many of these were not necessarily realised at the time. None the less, it is through later reflections that I have recognised the ways in which they affected the way that I think about the body. I have written elsewhere (Wellard 2009, 2013) about the significance of my early childhood experiences of physical activity and how growing up for periods of time in

Australia appeared to foster a greater orientation towards sport and outdoor physical activities. If I think about my time in Australia, I find it hard to get beyond images of being outside, playing on the beach, swimming in the sea and jumping off rocks into the water. Although these are distorted memories, in the Sartrean (Sartre 1956) sense, they are nevertheless significant in a number of ways. That they are my predominant memories, or ones that I choose to remember, suggests that they did have a bearing on my later orientation to sport and my body. During those times my body was something to be enjoyed and my whole being was unconsciously and unquestionably associated with a moving, experiencing body—a body that could feel the burning sand scorching my feet and even on some occasions it was so hot that it was difficult to place one's foot down for very long. A towel or blanket on the sand provided relief and I can remember thinking that if I ran fast my feet need not touch the ground and I could actually fly from my towel to the sea. The sea was, however, exciting: although it was enticing, it was also scary and the scariness made it even more exciting. It could sometimes suck me under and feel so strong that I felt completely helpless and I would have to battle to get back to the surface. Even though I can remember on many occasions thinking about how swimming in the sea was both dangerous and exciting, I was able to sum up the risks and make an appropriate decision about whether or not to return to the water.

In my early adolescence, I made choices about my body in ways that I could not really fully understand but I was, nevertheless, aware of making those choices. In many cases, I was making decisions by myself because I would often go to the beach on my own. On other occasions, when I was with friends, there were other considerations. I can remember having one friend who was not a strong swimmer and we made compromises about where we swam and what activities we did. The beaches where we played were also quite remote and were quite popular with surfers. Not the surfers who belonged to organised lifesaving clubs found in cities and more populated beaches, but 'hippie' surfers (or lifestyle surfers in the way that Wheaton [2004] describes). Often these surfers would be in groups when they were not in the water and would be drinking, smoking and most often sunbathing naked. This seemed completely natural to me and, at the time, I never had any cause to question this.

Looking back, it is reasonable to claim that those experiences did have a significant effect on my understanding of the body as something that was free to move around and be active. At the same time, it also fostered a much more casual approach to how I believed a body could be presented to others. My healthiness allowed me to be blind to an unhealthy body and when 'inconveniences', such as a broken arm or ruptured appendix, did occur they were not considered in terms of ill-health, but rather interruptions that were not permanent and could be manoeuvred around.

However, although health was not problematic, sport participation was not always plain sailing. My return to the UK in my early teens provided a stark contrast to those much more liberal embodied experiences on the beaches in Australia. I became conscious of how my body might not always conform, whether or not through a combination of a colder climate, a moral school curriculum, expectations in relation to gender performance and the dilemmas of dealing with a body that was changing physically and emotionally. Relating these to the expectations, phobias and paranoias of other bodies that were negotiating similar physiological and social changes consequently made my mid-teens, like for most others, fraught with anxieties and I felt obliged to maintain constant surveillance over what my body and other bodies were doing. Although sports remained an important part of my life, it was changing in the way that I could experience it. The only opportunities to experience the thrill of movement that I experienced on the beaches in Australia were to be found in more organised and rules-based traditional sports. The relative lack of restrictions and surveillance I experienced on the beaches in Australia was replaced by play and sporting activities that were heavily scrutinised and monitored by others, such as teachers or adults, and in public spaces by local authorities. In other words, what I could do with my body seemed markedly constrained and determined by others.

From an external perspective, my childhood and teenage years presented a time when I did engage in what might be considered a 'healthy lifestyle'. Physical activity was a key part of my everyday activities and something that I wanted to do. It was not something that my parents made me do and I never had any inclination that I was doing these activities to achieve health. During those times I never had cause to think about being unhealthy; health and unhealthiness did not enter the equation and were therefore not problematic, precisely because of my lack of awareness of it as an issue anyway. My complacency about being healthy and active was troubled only when after leaving school and feeling uncertain about a career path; rather than go to university I decided to get a job. After spending about a year working in uninspiring trainee jobs in London, I decided to train as a registered nurse. I had no clear rationale for doing this other than that I hated the idea of remaining in a 9-to-5 job and that I harboured a vague fascination for helping others in some way.

Even though I remained for only just over two of the three-year training course, the experience was a revelation for me in so many different ways. Until then I had not realised how naive I was about the human body, a body that could be ill, bleed, defecate, vomit and die. My experiences of nursing awakened an awareness of embodied existence—not that I could actually articulate these experiences fully but I was suddenly thrown into an 'enfleshed' (Woodward 2015) world where the body was presented to me in an alternative way. However, this new knowledge was not just about the physiological symptoms or conditions that necessitated a body to be placed in a hospital, but also about trying to understand the experience of an unhealthy person within the context of a social space of a ward in a hospital and in wider social terms. It was about trying to comprehend the contrasting identities of being a patient or a nurse, doctor or caregiver. I recognised myself as a symbol of a healthy body placed in a position that was almost diametrically opposed to the position of the patient in the bed. There were so many questions with which I struggled and I was particularly aware of the position of a patient who was, on the one hand, an individual (with a subjective life history and a range of physical and emotional needs) and, on the other, in this specific space a physical body with a condition to be treated. There were many contradictions. I could leave the ward, I could come and go and the only restriction on my movement related to my contractual hours in my role as a nurse. The freedom of movement that I had contrasted to that of a patient confined to a specific space, either a bed or the ward. This sudden restriction on the body, determined through the imposed identity of 'patient', raised questions (for me) about freedom and control and a contested body. Predictably, this type of philosophical questioning was not necessarily conducive to the operational role of a pragmatic nurse and it was, ultimately, questions such as these that made me reconsider nursing as my vocation. However, it galvanised my determination to study 'the social body' in more detail and sociology appeared to offer a way to do this.

More recently, because I have been grappling with issues relating to the embodied self and the ways in which the body is contemplated (in a multi-dimensional corporeal sense), reflective processes have become more prominent and, as such, I have felt a greater need to consider the relevance of my own experiences within my research activities. As Knowles and Gilbourne (2010) suggest, critical social science encourages an understanding of the self in a wider world context and, through an approach such as auto-ethnography, requires the author to engage in varying degrees of reflection. Consequently, in an attempt to step a little outside of my theoretical and methodological comfort zones and question further some of the issues relating to physical activity and its embodied experiences, I have attempted to apply an auto-ethnographical lens to my existing techniques. To the seasoned auto-ethnographer my attempts might be considered fairly rudimentary. However, my intention has not been to make claims that what follows in this book is an auto-ethnographic account of experiences of participating in an intensive period of physical training, but rather an attempt to incorporate a broader lens to existing 'tried and tested' techniques and be able to reflect on the complex social relationships that such an encounter reveals. To an extent, I have incorporated elements of more established retrospective ethnographic procedures (Sparkes 2002), as well as experience as it occurs by acknowledging emotional ethnography (Owen 2006) and experiential ethnography (Allen-Collinson 2014), so that a broader 'embodied ethnography' can be utilised.

Much of the appeal of auto-ethnographic writing has been in its ability to use 'loss' as a focus, particularly the notion of physical loss, and as a result this has created the need to shift the gaze inwards (Sparkes 1996, Ellis & Bochner 2000). In these cases, the social construction of 'otherness' or 'outsiderness' can be highlighted because it can capture the subjective individual experience of, for instance, being an outsider or becoming an outsider. Similarly, the subjective accounts of an individual experiencing a specific social activity are informative, such as the way that Delamont (2005) can describe taking part in capoeira and demonstrate the way she developed strategies to blend in, but had to remain constantly aware of her difference because of her gender, age and body type. Although issues relating to loss and outsiderness are not the central concerns within this research, an auto-ethnographical lens is considered worthwhile because it offers an insight into the processes of internalisation of the social body and how this is subjectively negotiated by individuals; as such, this provides a valuable contribution to any attempts to understand the social world.

Although the 'evidence' in this book draws from a range of sources, the central guiding point has been the material that I generated during my experiences taking part in an intensive programme of strength and conditioning training. This period of training required the services of a personal trainer or 'coach' over a period of eight months and my subsequent embracing of all things 'CrossFit' during this period and after. More recently, health issues related to undergoing surgery on my eyes has undoubtedly affected my thinking during this process. Ultimately, all of this has shaped the course of the book. At the same time, the interest in sport and the body that I have maintained throughout my life has also been developed in previous academic research. I have consciously attempted to incorporate the ideas generated in my previous research activities so that I could critically reflect further on the ideas that emerged then, and apply them in the light of experiences during the CrossFit training.

In as much as the personal narratives that inform my thinking are subjective, I consider that the ideas that arise from them are already 'out there' and not necessarily to be considered as new—rather the themes presented in this book are offered as additional to existing thought. What I am suggesting is, therefore, that the themes discussed can apply to all of us in some way, in a collective sense. In doing so, the book also sets out to challenge simplistic assumptions that the individual is a unique being, one that is constantly presented by contemporary neoliberal discourses as being in control of one's destiny and free to determine one's actions. Much of the background theory to the ideas generated in this book have been influenced by what might be explained as a contemporary version of existentialism, where individuality is connected within a social context in which freedom is inextricably connected to social responsibility. Subsequent formulations of power relationships are considered via Foucault, post-structuralism and embodied reflexivity.

Although the reflections above might be considered slightly over-indulgent for a traditional sociologist, they are included as a mechanism for generating questions. A reflexive approach is considered essential when exploring some of the issues relating to our understanding of a 'sporty' or 'healthy' body, especially as it is often the case that these two terms are conflated. It may be worthwhile, at this stage, offering a brief explanation of my methodological position that I have outlined previously:

> In terms of generating understanding about broader society, I am less interested in myself as a focus, unless it is as part of a reflexive approach to the development of the research questions or the methodological decision making. As Plummer states, 'the starting point is always the social' (Plummer 2010: 18) and, as a consequence, social research is about others and finding out about how other people have formed and constructed knowledge and ways to interact with others. This simplistic theoretical and methodological starting point was a reason that I was attracted to sociology in the first place. I had ideas that I had developed about myself and my place within society and these had generated many questions. However, I felt that I needed to explore the lives of other people (individuals and groups) in order to reassess those questions. At the same time, the intention underlying my research was to reassure myself that I was not living in a vacuum of my own thoughts, as I had presumed that it was more likely that my thinking was not unique. So, in order to answer questions, I needed to 'observe' the world and focus upon 'others'. As such, I have only considered myself important in terms of my reflexive contribution to the research process, both in terms of my theoretical and methodological position

(Bourdieu & Wacquant 1992). Consequently, my theoretical starting point is embedded in attempts to observe or engage with an empirical reality where acknowledging the subjective in terms of the reflexive stance of the researcher within the research process is crucial.

(Wellard 2013, p. 5)

Subsequent later experiences in adulthood of injury and illness, time spent as a patient and undergoing surgery, the physical and emotional aspects of these processes, 'being' a patient and placing my body in the hands of others, contribute to my thought processes. All of this assists in my attempts to understand how the subjective might influence general understanding of what healthy means at different times and in different circumstances. Importantly, this also provides an interesting, as well as complimentary, information source that is generated through previous knowledge developed in other roles, such as a nurse, teacher and sports coach.

In terms of organised physical activities, for most of my life, tennis and swimming have been my major sporting pastimes. I have always liked doing other things, but these two sports tended to take priority. However, throughout my life I have 'trained' my body in some way, whether this has been in terms of going to the gym or doing training that involved drills, cardio and flexibility. I have never considered myself a sports fanatic, although I imagine many of my friends and work colleagues would say that I am. Nevertheless, sport is a big part of my life or, rather, physical activity as well as sport are a big part of my life. In recent years, however, health-related problems with my eyesight have meant that I have not been able to play tennis in the way that I have done in the past or would like to continue to do so. This has meant that I have been playing less and have been consciously looking for other activities to fill the gap. Going to the gym has, therefore, become one of the ways in which I have been able to fill this gap.

Serendipity

Although my early sporting identity had been formed through tennis and swimming, as mentioned above in more recent years my failing eyesight has contributed to an increased participation in gym-related activities. Although I cannot physically 'see' a tennis ball as well as I used to and continuing to play has highlighted my 'inability' to do so, going to the gym has been less problematic, in that there is far less emphasis on sight (and focusing on a fast moving ball). I describe in more detail how going to the gym fits in with my lifestyle and my changing body in terms of the way in which I am able to engage with physical activity in my book on *Sport, Fun and Enjoyment* (Wellard 2013). However, I realised that because I was embracing working out at the gym more and tennis no longer held the same appeal that it had before (because of the way that I was able to engage in it), I found that fitness training in the gym was becoming my 'sport' of choice. In December 2014, when I was putting together the initial ideas for this book, my department at work introduced a range of strength and conditioning sessions (as part of an overhaul of activities that they were able to provide for students and the general public). I thought I would take advantage of one of these, a series of personal training sessions based on Olympic lifting and weight-lifting techniques. These were one-to-one sessions designed to look at and improve form and technique in strength movements as well as physical activities to incorporate into training programmes for sport. These sessions continued until the summer of 2015. During this time, I became aware that my trainer (as well as her partner) was heavily involved in CrossFit. Until then I did not really know much about CrossFit. However, further investigation revealed that it was an activity developed from cross-training practices and, in particular, elements of gymnastics, weight training and aerobic fitness. It is probably not surprising that I responded well to the sessions bearing in mind that I had engaged in many of these activities in various forms throughout my life and have always enjoyed fitness-related activities. Consequently, when my trainer started to incorporate the core activities found in CrossFit, I was curious to find out more. As I started to learn more about the correct techniques and form required for Olympic lifting, my enthusiasm to embrace CrossFit increased much more than I expected when I first started the personal training sessions. At the same time, a colleague of mine had also started to engage in CrossFit but in a much more serious fashion. In his case, he had started to participate in a local 'box' and had embraced what could be considered a CrossFit identity.

On a personal level, I was enjoying the one-to-one aspects of personal training and engaging in the gym in ways that I had not done before. At that time, however, I did not feel the need to subscribe wholeheartedly to CrossFit. From my initial investigations, I also had reservations about CrossFit in general—in particular, what seemed like an exclusivity that it projected. It did seem to me that in the UK most participants were very much more serious weight trainers in their mid to late 20s who had been engaging in lifting weights and gym training but were looking for something more exclusive. It is here that the appeal of CrossFit lies, in that it provides a form of recognisable sporting identity. For instance, there is a significant difference between someone identifying as, for example, a rugby player or a tennis player compared with a 'gym-goer'. A rugby or tennis player presents a specific 'image' that one can perfect and present. This appears to be very much part of the appeal of CrossFit because it does convey a specific identity. Consequently, like many other sports, most of my reservations have been about how someone of my age (in my 50s) could fit in.

It was at this stage that I was 'passed on' to the partner of the member of staff who was taking the training sessions. He was already involved in CrossFit and had qualified as a CrossFit coach as well as having a background in strength and conditioning training. He had also taken part in several competitions and told me that there were masters divisions in these competitions, and that I had potential to do well in them. Consequently, the experience of taking part in the initial introductory sessions and the exposure to a new form of fitness training offered possibilities for further investigation

Before the sessions offered at work I had always thought that gym-based personal training was an interesting phenomenon, particularly from a sociological perspective, in terms of its relationship to a highly commercialised 'fitness industry' in the way that Pronger (2002) describes. As a result of this, I have generally considered personal training to differ from traditional sports coaching, and it is only more recently that I have had cause to consider why I had developed these views. Although I had always valued the coaching I received in tennis, either on a one-to-one basis or as part of a team, my understanding of coaching was based on recognition of the skills and expertise possessed by the coaches who guided me. I had not always been so convinced about the capabilities of the personal trainers whom I have seen at the gyms I have attended, and this undoubtedly influenced subsequent deliberations about whether I could trust placing 'my body in their hands'. In the case of the sessions offered at work, however, I knew that the person who was running the sessions was a very capable trainer and educator, with a substantial background in sport and exercise training and strength and conditioning. By mentioning this, I suggest that, before one gets to the stage of taking part in any form of personal training activity, there are many important considerations to be made. Here, the notion of trust and the recognition of the dynamics of a one-to-one encounter highlight some of the complex relationships that operate in such situations. It is not simply a case of 'going to the gym' or 'getting a personal trainer', but having to negotiate a series of social encounters that offer a range of contrasting outcomes. These relationships are very much what Foucault (1980) talks about when he describes relationships of power. These are power relationships not governed by forms of simple dominance where one individual has power over another, but ones that are much more complex and dynamic. A session with a personal trainer provides a good example, precisely because it highlights the forms of power that not only operate between participants but also are influenced by a range of competing social discourses generated about the body, health, fitness, age, ability, consumer culture and so much more.

From the outset, I found that I really enjoyed the sessions. They were a combination of instruction and practice, along with some intensive workouts. I liked being physically 'pushed' and relished the serious focus, in particular being in a learning situation. I relished exploring the capabilities of my body and being guided by another person in routines and exercises that I had subconsciously (or probably consciously) avoided when training on my own. At the same time, I enjoyed the subtle forms of power relationships that I mention above, where I was the one that had to follow the lead and be told what to do. It was a welcome contrast to the expected 'leadership' that my academic role demanded. It was similar to the way in which I enjoy having opportunities to listen to a lecture rather than presenting one. The sessions, therefore, embraced a range of physical and social experiences and allowed me to feel comfortable putting myself 'in the hands' of the trainer. The important point here is that in these circumstances, and within this context, I am complicit in this relationship of power and allow myself at times to be subservient because I recognise that I have something to gain from this exchange. I am, however, aware of the subjectivity in these accounts of my experiences. However, my subjectivity is understood alongside the many other forms of relationships that are forged within the context of many other gym spaces and settings where those engaging enter with different expectations and motivations. In these cases, other factors might be more significant, such as losing weight or the personal trainer's perception of clients as sources of potential income. Nevertheless, the point is that these relationships *are* subjective and open to interpretation and, consequently, need to be recognised as such before we can attempt to understand further the complexities of contemporary health and fitness pursuits (and, indeed, embodied wellbeing).

Whose body is it anyway?

To investigate some of the questions that I have raised above, I felt that it would be instructive to engage in CrossFit at a much greater level. This was so that I could not only experience and assess the embodied aspects of taking part in an intensive period of strength and conditioning training, but also explore those reservations that I had about embracing an activity that was not specifically aimed at an older body. Consequently, the core material that I draw on throughout this book is taken from a diary (in the form of a blog) that charted my experiences between September 2015 and March 2016. The specific goal of the training in terms of the remit for my coach was to 'get' my body into the appropriate levels of physical fitness to be able to take part in the 2016 CrossFit Open, and attempt to qualify for the regional heats of the CrossFit Games. This goal provided the focus for the training and established a concrete goal for my coach to develop a training programme. However, the intention was also to explore the embodied experiences of 'doing' an intensive period of physical activity and, subsequently, to attempt to understand, in more depth, the range of personal, social, psychological and physical factors that undoubtedly contribute to engaging in such an activity.

In order to explore the issues introduced above I have structured the book into the following chapters. Rather than follow a conventional process, where an initial review of the literature is explored, I felt that it was important to introduce some of the 'story' first so that a more detailed discussion can be read in better context. What follows in this book is a series of diary entries that detail my experiences as I progress through this training period. The intention is that, by detailing what happened, I provide a foundation upon which to reflect on the thoughts and experiences generated during this period, and then explore them in more theoretical detail.

Chapter 2 introduces the period of training by incorporating a series of my initial reflections as I started the training programme. My experiences presented several anticipated themes as well as many that were unexpected. Most noticeably, the emerging story reveals much about the physical experience of the body being put through intensive exercise, noticeably in terms of pleasure and pain, as well as other socio-cultural 'issues' relating to relationships of power, trust and the role of 'expert' health advisor. The discussion in Chapter 2 provides the opportunity to consider the themes that emerged during the training period in greater theoretical detail.

Chapter 3 applies the themes that emerged to explore questions relating to social understanding of the role of 'personal trainers' and how they fit into current formulations of a health practitioner and commercial entrepreneur. In addition, I consider the complex power relationships at large for all parties involved in any fitness-related training. The chapter concludes with an overview of how embodied thinking can assist in our understanding of health and fitness.

Chapter 4 provides further diary entries relating to the embodied aspects of engaging in fitness-related pursuits. Here, themes relate to the notion of a healthy versus an unhealthy body, the pleasures to be found in what can be considered 'adult' play and the contrasting ways in which pain and suffering are managed. Chapter 5 explores the themes in Chapter 4 in more detail—in particular, using an embodied approach, contemporary constructions of health, pleasure and pain are considered while bearing in mind the complexity and subjectivity of the context of engagement and the impact of the individuals taking part (whether training participant, trainer or spectator). The chapter explores further the experiences of pain and pleasure in physical activity pursuit. Providing examples of pain and pleasure that are not necessarily experienced uniformly—and may be perceived as opposite by many others—highlights the complexity of making assertions about the merits or not of a particular activity.

Chapter 6 provides further diary reflections. In this case it highlights the significance of the broader appeal of a particular sporting identity. My experiences taking part in CrossFit not only entailed a heavy physical commitment to the training, but also required me to learn the discourses of having a CrossFit identity.

Chapter 7 develops these ideas further by incorporating the notion of bodies moving into physical and social spaces, where the body is 'given over' to the overarching expectations of what bodies should do in a particular space, as well as the roles they might have. The discussion here can be compared with the themes explored in Chapter 3 and highlights how the 'knowledge' and expertise expected from established health professionals (such as doctors and nurses) is replicated in the 'gym/exercise' space, where the established experts are the gym instructor, coaches and personal trainers. The chapter uses my experiences of undergoing fitness training as a mechanism to explore these similarities—chiefly how the body is complicit in acts of subservience and obedience. At the same time, it reveals the significant elements of acquiring a social identity through the description of my 'metamorphosis' into a legitimate CrossFitter. In doing so the chapter explores further the notion of identity and the extent to which we have 'control' over our identity(ies).

Chapter 8 provides some 'final thoughts' and attempts to draw together the key themes generated in this book. It draws on the themes described in the previous chapters in order to consider the way we think about the body within the context of health, wellbeing and sport. Consequently, it reveals some of the limitations of current approaches to thinking about the body—in terms of not only the way that we theorise the body, but also the way that we seek to explore the body. In doing so an appeal is made for more reflective, embodied investigation, analysis and theoretical explanation of the body.

2

BEING TRAINED

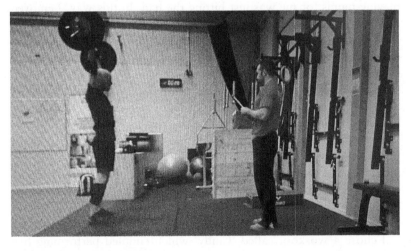

FIGURE 2.1 Ian and coach JP

August 2015—getting ready

My personal training sessions had finished at the beginning of July, which meant that for the rest of that month and throughout August I was continuing training on my own. As I knew that I was going to start the more intensive programme in September I have more motivation and I was keen to practise some of the techniques I have been taught so that I was ready to start.

Although at this stage I'm still undecided about CrossFit, nevertheless because the training is very much geared towards getting me ready to actually compete then I did need to practise some of the specific routines. Part of this was to engage in workouts of the day (WoDs). These are intensive routines usually consisting of a range of activities that are either timed or carried out within a certain amount of time. The intention with these workouts is to record either the time taken or the number of rounds that were performed to provide an indication of, I suppose, performance. In relation to the CrossFit Games detailed recording of times and performance is really important and as I was training towards being able to qualify I obviously needed to get into the habit of monitoring my performance.

I think this is where the period of training is going to be really interesting, precisely because of my reservations about putting myself in a situation where I have to compete with and against others. It's not that I've never done that before as tennis like any other traditional sport is built around competition. I have competed in numerous tennis events in both singles and doubles and I think it was always a love–hate relationship with this aspect. If I'm being really honest, the best part of playing tennis for me was just hitting the ball. In this way, I enjoyed drilling the ball for hours on end in practice sessions much more than I did the competitions. As I got older the appeal of competing has diminished even more. However, I still really like the idea of pushing myself so this is where my fascination with personal training, strength and conditioning training and, indeed, CrossFit has developed because of the elements within these activities that cater towards pushing the body and forms of individual, personal activity.

So, today after doing what seems like lots of practice, I thought I would put myself to the test and do my first proper WoD—on my own. I had already done some variations of these workouts with my trainer and her partner. It was interesting that these have been introduced into the sessions at an early stage, before I even knew about CrossFit. Later on it became clear the purpose of these activities.

I chose a workout called 'Cindy' which entailed performing five pullups, 10 press-ups and 15 squats. Each of these is performed in succession and constitutes one round. Within this session, the intention is to perform as many rounds as possible in the space of 20 minutes. I thought that this workout would be useful as I knew that I could do each of the activities fairly easily, but what I really wanted to experiment with was doing these over a period of 20 minutes in a sustained fashion and having the chance to think about pacing myself as well as pushing myself—in particular on my own and without somebody encouraging me. It would also provide a benchmark that I could record and compare with when I did it again in the future. At the same time I wanted to experience pushing my body and the associated physical feelings that would emerge from this exertion. I think what has been really interesting in the past months has been learning about physical pain and exertion and pushing myself through it. I have done this before in other sports but then again it is different because, for instance, in a game like tennis even though you may be pushing yourself physically there are always rest periods and it is not necessarily continuous for 20 minutes. However, there are other activities that I have taken part in such as quite high intensity aerobic sessions that I did in my early 20s. Nevertheless, it never gets any easier when you are in an activity and your body starts to scream out at you stop and you can feel yourself panting and sweating and your heart racing because as a pragmatic part of the self says you shouldn't really be doing this anymore. So, experiencing these feelings is important and important to capture and reflect upon.

I made sure that I had a stopwatch and a piece of paper next to it with 1–15 written in a row so that I could tick off each round as I finished it. Before starting I had considered how many rounds it was likely that I could do. It was difficult to really know what I could do but I thought that 10 was probably a good guide. I then added a few more just in case. When I started I was very much aware of pacing myself and did not want to go into it hell for leather. I thought beforehand that five pullups will be really easy, 10 press-ups would also be easy and then the 15 squats will provide a time for recovery. My predictions were correct. I purposefully tried to keep a steady pace and as I completed each round I ticked off the number on the paper. I tried not to look at the stopwatch too much but at 10 minutes I noted that I'd done eight rounds already. I think this was a bit of a mistake because when I realise that I was halfway through and I had already reached eight I knew that I was going to be able to do 10 without any problem. So, I think that rather than pushing myself more it made me relax and while I was getting tired, the thought that I was going to reach my target might have stopped me from pushing myself harder. So while I continued for the 20 minutes I don't think the second half was as intense as the first half. Nevertheless I managed to do 14 rounds and was pretty pleased with this. This was a really useful learning curve and although I was shattered at the end of it I know that I was not as exhausted as I have been in some of the other sessions that had been led by my trainer.

First week of programme

I have now officially started my training. I had the first session on Saturday and the intention is that I have one formal training session with my trainer (coach JP) at the start of the week and he will then provide me with an outline of the sessions that I need to do during the week. Before I describe what happened on that first session, I think I need to say that there is so much going on in terms of actually what I am experiencing that I really need to organise my thoughts and the subsequent posts that I make in this blog. Consequently, what I will attempt to do over the next few weeks is give a description of what happens in the sessions that I have with coach JP but not necessarily focus always on the specific detail. Because there appear to be so many themes emerging, I will attempt to concentrate on a particular theme in one post rather than throwing them all in getting a bit confused.

Although I have already had some sessions with coach JP they were more like one-off sessions. This session, however, did feel like it was the start of something more meaningful. Maybe more so because I had in the back of my mind (well maybe not the back of my mind as it appeared to be quite a central thought) that I was really committing myself to something. This suggested to me that there were various other factors at play that, in turn, had implications on how I was going to experience the training. These were factors that had not necessarily been the case or so apparent when I have been going to the gym on my own or just having a one-off session with a personal trainer. Recognition of a 'commitment' meant that I was not only setting out on something that just related to me but it also meant that I was committing myself to others in terms of their expectations and the work that they were going to do with me. In coach JP's case, there was also something at stake in his commitment to training me as well as what he could get out of the 'project'—in that I was in some ways his guinea pig in terms of him gaining experience training an older adult. Awareness of all of this created a sense of trepidation and a feeling of nervousness in terms of what I was letting myself in for but at the same time there was a level of excitement at the thought of getting involved in something that was going to be a legitimate and meaningful period of training.

In my first post I mentioned about my early perceptions of CrossFit and while I'm still not sure the extent to which I will ultimately embrace it, there is clearly something seductive about the identity and being able to adopt something that does have, or is beginning to establish, an identity of its own as a 'sport'. I think this has resonance with my life at the moment, particularly because of the way in which my sporting identity as a tennis player is very much on the wane.

All of this stuff is going on even before I get to the stage of actually doing some physical activity. But I can't ignore that, because it clearly affects the way in which I approach the activity. It is not just about me doing some physical exercises; there are some much more existential questions operating and influencing the way I feel now and will undoubtedly affect how I experience the next few months. Whether I can detail all of these is another matter, but I want to have a go at experiencing this in its broadest sense.

Saturday session

The session started off with coach JP asking me a series of questions about previous injuries and operations. This was in an attempt to get a picture of my physical body and how any previous injuries or surgery may have impacted upon or, indeed, may affect my movement and performance in the exercises that are core to CrossFit. It is always interesting in these situations when one has to talk about one's body as a form of 'other'—in some ways it is like a process of separating oneself from one's own physical body and this becomes more apparent in the techniques that we have to actually detail and account for as a history of the physical body, or an individual's body. Things like mapping out a history of injury, or taking physical measurements are pretty much part and parcel of most sports and sports training—and CrossFit is no exception. But what is interesting for me is actually thinking about this process and having the feeling that my life or 'me' is being mapped out and encapsulated on a piece of paper or in a computer document. Then, assessments and conclusions are being formed about the details of how a subsequent exercise plan can be developed. It's very much like a patient going into hospital where an initial analysis is made, a subsequent diagnosis followed by a course of treatment. This suggests there are some interesting relationships that are being formed and in particular a high level of trust along with commitment by all parties to adhere to the prescribed treatment. With this trust there is a high amount of complicity with all parties needing to 'be on board' for it to work.

Right, I said I wasn't going to try to analyse things too much to start with but it is difficult precisely because there is so much going on. Thus, something really simple like detailing a previous injury history prompts many thoughts about the implication and meaning of doing this. I will, no bounds, come back to this many times in subsequent posts. In the meantime, after we had had a discussion about injuries and had attempted to establish what our goals were, we started with the physical stuff. The intention was for the sessions that I did with coach JP to be about developing technique, practising movements and gradually increasing core strength and flexibility. We started off with some general warm-ups and this was followed by some instruction about basic Olympic lifting and squatting techniques. Nevertheless, although this was an instruction/learning element of the session it was still physically tiring as it included a series of repetitions of the movements (such as thrusters and squats). In the overall scheme of things, however, it was meant as just a 'warm-up' for the main WoD. In this case, coach JP had devised a workout that he called a 9/11. The intention was for it to not only be a workout but also provide a benchmark for my performance in subsequent WoDs. This was important as performances in WoDs were always recorded in some form or other, whether in terms of how many rounds could be completed within a set time or the overall time taken to complete the specific activities within the WoD.

For this activity, I had to complete the following rounds:

1.   400-metre run
2.   11 thrusters (with a 30-kg bar)
3.   11 box steps
4.   11 chin-up burpees
5.   11 front squats (30-kg bar)
6.   11 shoulder thrusts (30-kg bar)
7.   11 clean and jerks (30-kg bar)
8.   11 deadlifts (30-kg bar)
9.   400-metre run

When looking at the activities on paper and taking them at face value they look pretty innocuous. However, doing them in one go is another matter. I suppose it is the case of putting the theory into practice and, even though I don't want to make distinctions between the two, it is sometimes hard to really predict what is going to happen, and in this case to the body. It might be the case that when one looks at the activities on paper it is easy to isolate each exercise and think oh yes I can easily do the 400-metre run or 11 thrusters. However, doing them one after another and being conscious of a clock ticking makes it exhausting in a range of ways because halfway through I was really aware of voices screaming out to me you need to stop. These were voices from my heart telling me that I needed to slow down because it was pumping too fast. In fact the voices didn't need to tell me as I could feel it and hear it thumping inside my rib cage. And speaking of my rib cage, there seemed to be a clamp fixed all the way round it, tightening every second. I could feel my head throbbing and I was sweating. I know that everybody sweats, but I'm also aware that generally I don't break into a sweat very much. I can sometimes play tennis for several hours and not really sweat, especially compared to the way that I was doing so after only a couple minutes. I could also feel that my face was turning a puce colour. Although I didn't have a mirror I could actually sense by the heat that I was feeling in my skin that it probably looked that colour.

In addition to the physical reactions to performing these exercises, there were also voices in my head screaming at me you should stop. There must be some part of the brain that houses a logical room where there are a number of 'Mr Spocks' who are voicing their concerns about what the rest of the body is doing and sending out messages that this is all illogical. However, despite all of this, there is something else happening that is making me continue and override all of these alarm calls. It helps that coach JP is encouraging me and telling me that it will hurt but it is okay to push on. Not wanting to let him down or for him to see me as someone who gives up, I carry on. I also don't want to let myself down. So there must be some aspect in my psyche that operates in terms of a motivational speaker. This makes me think (although I didn't think it at the time) that there is some aspect of 'letting go' that cannot really be explained fully through conventional interpretations of going into a 'zone'. However there does seem to be a sense that there is a need to overcome all the panic alarms that the body is signalling to me, through the physical feeling of the tightness of my chest and the clamping of my body—as well as all the thoughts that are being vividly expressed inside my head (Are you mad? Why are you doing this on Saturday morning?). I am obviously conscious enough to be aware of these thoughts and these physical feelings. However, there is a big BUT: I'm still enjoying it in a strange way. I can't really pinpoint exactly how I'm enjoying this at the moment and where this enjoyment is derived from. The physical reactions to the exertions are not pleasurable but I am aware of wanting to push myself further and wanting to complete the task. These feelings are able to dominate or override all those other physical reactions and negative thoughts.

I'm also aware that I'm enjoying being coached. I trust coach JP and I think his enthusiasm is infectious. In some ways I'm also surprised by what I can do and may be this is an indication of how I may have set my expectations lower and maybe I need to consider why I have done this.

I finish the WoD and coach JP notes down the time. It took me just over 16 minutes to do, so that means I have set down a benchmark for subsequent 'assessments' of my body. I don't really have any way to make comparisons with other times because this is an activity that coach JP has devised himself. However, it will provide an indication of progress when I repeat this further down the line. That is the idea, although I haven't really thought about what it will be like if I go slower the next time.

One of the big themes here is related to the experience of pain. In this particular case, and thinking about how I have described the activity above, the word pain does not really adequately describe those experiences. It wasn't pain in the way that I generally understand it in terms of comparing it with the pain that I felt when I injured my knee a couple of years ago or maybe a sharp stabbing pain in a particular area of the body—or indeed the throbbing pain of a migraine. In these particular cases the use of 'pain' as a descriptor provides a reasonable mechanism to convey to someone else what the feeling is like. The sensations I experienced during the workout seem to me to be more usefully described in terms of an intensive exhaustion. It was an exhaustion that affected my entire body, emotionally and physically. I want to explore this aspect in the coming weeks.

Tuesday session

The next session was one of two that I needed to carry out on my own during the week. Coach JP had set out the routines and I was to do them and then record the times in each of the WoDs at the end of each session. For this session I had to perform a series of warm-ups and then a series of conditioning and technique activities, which included doing several rounds of front squats, thrusters, push presses, and back squats. These were actually quite exhausting but were meant as a general warm-up before the final WoD.

The main WoD was a succession of burpees and kettlebell swings (30/15/9) which were to be performed as fast as possible and the overall time recorded.

I noticed, on this occasion, that it was a little more difficult working out on my own, especially in terms of getting myself ready to do the timed WoD. I think that as I was fairly tired after doing the initial warm-ups there was almost a sense of foreboding about the final WoD in that I was aware of the need to time it—and this presented a fear of failure in that I might actually do this really slowly. Logically, this was pretty silly as I didn't know what time was a good time or a bad time in the first place. However, it didn't stop me from worrying about doing it really slowly.

I also noticed the difference between the Saturday session where coach JP had been able to pace out the activities and my sense of compliance with what he was saying and asking me to do, whereas, on my own, I was aware of my own input and a slight concern about not doing it 'properly'. I found that just before the start of the final

WoD, and when I set up the timer it took me a long time to get started. I kept dithering when it came to pressing the timer start. In the end I got slightly annoyed with myself and pressed it making myself go to it straightaway.

Once again, my perceptions before the activity were not the same as the experiences of doing it. I had initially thought the kettlebell swings would be more tiring but it was the other way round. Indeed, doing 30 burpees in a row was really taxing and it seemed like I had to take an extended catch of breath before I started the 30 kettlebell swings. It may have been because these seemed easier in comparison to the burpees—it gave me a little bit of a boost. The numbers factor came into it again because after completing 30 of each, doing 15 the next round seemed less daunting. There was, in fact, a lot of playing with numbers in my mind during these activities. It seems like setting targets and milestones will become a prominent factor in forthcoming exercise routines. For instance, in this case in the first round of 30 I felt a sense of urgency in terms of getting past 15 as that would provide a milestone to pass and also reassurance that the following round of 15 would be achievable. Consequently, there were many things going on in my head such as setting targets in the first round and then thinking about the overall WoD, trying to map out the whole activity and break it down into stages. I think one of the things that has become more apparent is the need to pace myself, not only in terms of my physical fitness when performing the activities but also in terms of the broader goals over the next few months.

Second week—lessons learnt (already)

I know that it is only early days but I feel that I have already learnt a lot—and not just about CrossFit and strength and conditioning training but also many other things relating to my own body capabilities and putting things in perspective. I do, however, feel a bit daft in that I have been doing exactly the things that I warn my new PhD students not to do when they first start their research—not to run before they can walk. I can hear myself telling them not to get carried away with thinking about the final end result and take time to get into the process. So, what have I been doing? Exactly the opposite—diving in head first, thinking about the final podium and achieving fastest times when I need to get myself, physically and mentally, into a state where I can possibly attempt to do that. I have now realised that I need to reign in those expectations and concentrate on gradually developing. Therefore, in this post, I think the main theme is about PACING in terms of both physically and mentally developing a better understanding of what the next months will involve and require from me.

As I mentioned in my last post, in the first week it hit me just what I had let myself in for and I think there was a kind of physical and mental reaction to this in terms of a feeling of physical exhaustion and mental fatigue or even a kind of panic. These feelings were exacerbated when I was doing the weekly sessions on my own and when I had more time to worry about all of these things on my own. So when it came round to the next session with coach JP on Saturday, I was feeling a little bit flat. However, it was really encouraging to chat through these things and be put through my paces again. It helped reaffirm to myself that I actually can do these things but also to be reassured that it was only the start and it was going to take time to develop, learn the techniques properly, and develop my overall fitness and strength. This is where it is so easy to get carried away beforehand and not put things into context. So while there was an understandable sense of excitement prior to training, I needed to actually get started to be able to recognise what the training actually involved and how it would affect my day-to-day life, probably in ways that I had been able to really predict.

So the idea of pace and learning to pace myself has been a valuable lesson this week, precisely because this applies to developing a better understanding of my physical capabilities. I suppose everybody does it when they think about taking up a different sport or activity—one makes assumptions about 'what I think I can do' and 'what I want it to do' before there is a recognition of what they actually can do. A lot of this is related to working out the limits of one's body not only in terms of what it can do during a particular session (such as how much weight can be lifted or how many pullups one can do) but also in terms of how much recovery the body needs. One thing that I'm trying to gauge at the moment is working out how much soreness and aching I can manage throughout the week. This is particularly in terms of learning about what are the types of pain that I can work through. Being aware of potential signs of longer-term injury is important and being able to adapt the training schedule. At the moment, the plan is to follow a one day on one day off schedule and something I have to learn about is following this but then also finding out what I can do on the day off. For example, last week I had a session with coach JP on Saturday and then he gave me session plans for the following Tuesday and Thursday. On the Sunday after the first session I felt a bit stiff and tired. However, on the Monday I felt okay and thought that I would do some gentle exercise at the gym on my own. So after I did the planned session on Tuesday, the next day I was really shattered and I think this contributed to my feeling of flatness and panic about the task at hand. So what I realised is that I needed to change my attitude to training and learn to be more focused upon the training plan and recognise it in terms of a gradual process over a period of time.

The lessons I have learnt about pacing not only relate to my recognition of what my physical body can do but are also combined with a mental recognition of the temporal pathway that I am undertaking. Simplistically, it is about keeping my emotions in check and not running before I can walk.

Mind games

I mentioned in a previous post that I wanted to talk more about the notion of mind games. The psychological elements of my training have been much more prominent than I envisaged when I started. Although I had expected there would be a lot going on in terms of how I could cope mentally (as well as physically) with the level of training period and also attempting to develop a CrossFit mind-set, the different ways in which the psychological factors have emerged have taken me somewhat by surprise. I have also noticed how these mind games operate both internally and externally. The games that I play in my own mind tend to take the form of constantly reassuring myself that I can continue, whether in a specific activity or the whole programme. They also emerge in terms of questions that I ask myself about my ability to be able to become proficient enough in all the activities required and whether my technical knowledge will be sufficient. However, in addition to the internal struggles there are mind games that are played out with others.

Internal struggles

There seem to be a range of games that are played out inside my head. Much of these are concerned with what could be considered as motivational talk and attempts to work out strategies that could help me complete a set workout. My mind plays a big part in convincing myself or my body that I can actually physically complete a session. These mind games end up becoming forms of operational strategies whereby I try to work out the best way to be able to complete the activity. For instance, if it is an activity where I have to do as many rounds as possible in a set period of time (such as 15 minutes) I have to work out in advance the best way that I can go about undertaking the challenge. This invariably means working out a rough estimate of how many rounds I might be able to do within the period and trying to work out a pacing strategy so that I am able to set out a realistic time plan. These are all pretty much straightforward thinking action plans; however, these mental strategies become much more important when a workout suggests to me that I might have difficulties doing it or something in my mind tells me that it is going to be hard or even impossible to do. These set up internal struggles whereby I have to evaluate and debate inside my head the best course of action. In some cases the internal turmoil about whether I can or cannot do the session is overridden when I actually get started. As it often seems to be the case that when I do get started the physical dimensions kick in and the mental aspects become much more related to a motivational role. However (and I mentioned it in an earlier post), about how overthinking before starting an activity can sometimes cause procrastination and added frustration. In a way it is like standing on the edge of a diving board and looking down and then hesitating. Rather than just getting on with it (and diving in), the delayed reaction and period of hesitation allow any (of the many) doubts to kick in. Being aware of this doesn't really help and ends up generating another mind game based around working out ways in which I can sidestep those initial feelings of doubt insecurity and fear of failure.

Others

Within the context of the CrossFit sessions it has become apparent that I'm also playing mind games with others. I mentioned before (in the post about suffering for my art) that I had become aware of the way in which I had to moderate the feedback that I give to coach JP. Although I try to be as honest as possible in terms of how I describe the way I'm feeling physically after a session or how I evaluate the amount of effort that I needed to put into an activity, I am aware that the information that I offer will be acted upon in various ways. So I have to decide whether the assessments I make of something like a routine which involves lifting heavy weights is actually a fair indication of what I can do and that my coach will understand my description in the same way that I do. Thus if I say something was pretty easy I have to be really sure that it was really easy because otherwise the way that coach JP would interpret my assessment would be that I could do more and the intensity level should be raised. While I really want to progress as much as I can, I still have to play around with the doubts and fears that I am pushing myself too much. Therefore, I am aware that there is an editing process, albeit a very fast one, when I do provide feedback. The same applies to my response to a question about how I am feeling in relation to whether I am sore after the previous day's session or have any specific pain. If I am asked this, I immediately deliberate upon what constitutes pain and end up plunging into an abyss of ontological conundrums.

Constant surveillance of the information that I provide to coach JP (apart from making me seem neurotic) not only is a result of the uncertainties that I have about my performances and whether I am 'making the grade', but also indicates an embodied awareness that is being informed by external technologies of (what) a 'CrossFit' body (should look and act like). Therefore, while I consider that the levels of trust formed between coach JP and myself within the context of a coach/athlete relationship are not in question, what is highlighted is the significance of forms of communication and the ways that meaning is interpreted. If I do not have a clear idea of how I am feeling and performing (physically and psychologically) then it becomes even more difficult for the coach to accurately understand progress. Maybe, a problem here is overthinking—but sometimes it is difficult not to.

Progress?

I have now completed three months of my training and because it is halfway through the planned six-month programme, it is a good time to reflect upon 'how I have been doing'. The notion of progress is, however, something that I am constantly thinking about but I find it difficult to fully recognise the extent of my progress—and that is presuming that there has been any. I've mentioned this before in other posts about how I find it difficult to actually gauge whether I am improving and maybe because this has more to do with the training drawing upon such a wide range of sporting practices and, consequently, there are a range of skills and movements that I have to develop. Nevertheless, I do think that in the last couple of weeks there have been some breakthrough 'moments' in my sessions with coach JP and he has commented about areas where he feels that I have made progress. This does offer a boost to my confidence in that it provides reassurance that I have made some strides forward although these affirmative signs are always played out against constant doubts in my mind about the enormity of the task, particularly in terms of how much I have to learn as well as re-educate my body. These apparent breakthroughs have made us consider that there is 'evidence' to suggest that I am improving. And it is this notion of evidence that I plan to consider further when I write up this research in more detail, particularly in terms of broader questions about assessment and measuring progression, not only from a coaching perspective but also from the point of view of the participant.

In the last two Friday coaching sessions, coach JP planned programmes that finished with the following WoDs:

1. A 12-minute WoD consisting of 7 hang snatches, 14 step ups and 5 back squats. In true 'drill-sergeant' fashion he told me that if I put the bar down at any stage, I would have to do 10 burpees.
2. 21, 15, 9 rounds of deadlift @ 40 kg and ring rows—with 7 burpees over the bar every minute on the minute.

I don't know whether the burpee elements were a psychological ruse, but they worked in that I was determined to complete the first WoD without putting the bar down and the second by making sure that I had to do as few as possible—by getting the task done quickly. In both cases, when I started I made sure that I settled into a steady pace and knuckled down to the task. I completed the WoD without having to put the bar down and found that I managed to do the 12 minutes relatively easily. For the second one, I only had to do the burpees three times as once again I had managed to settle into a steady rhythm. In our discussions afterwards, we were able to recognise that there had been definite progress in the way that I was now managing to pace myself better. It was also encouraging for me that, on both occasions, coach JP had overestimated the times I would take to complete the WoDs. In the first one, he had expected me to put the bar down at least once and, in the second, he had thought I would take much longer.

Consequently, the last few weeks have been a real boost to my confidence in that I can actually 'see' some form of improvement. This still has to be put into context in terms of the whole programme and the continued progress that I have to make if I want to have any chance of being able to be ready to attempt the qualifying rounds.

3

HEALTH AND FITNESS 'KNOWLEDGE'

Theorising (fitness) body-reflexive practices

Introduction

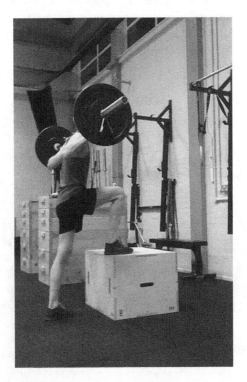

FIGURE 3.1   An activity in my training programme

In Chapter 2, I provided some reflections on my experiences during the initial stages of the training programme. Although they were obviously personal in terms of how I interpreted what was happening to me, in this chapter I explore the themes with a sociological lens so that I can incorporate the 'bigger picture' and attempt to understand the context of when, where and how these experiences were being lived. In doing so, I hope to highlight that my personal experiences can be read through broader embodied processes, which ultimately move beyond what may be considered a subjective experience in the first place. Figure 3.1 may help bring some of the reflections alive and provide an example of what I was doing for the reader. However, the context is understood with an acknowledgement that I am undergoing this training with a certain goal in mind and have formulated a specific understanding of the role of physical activity in contemporary society (through a personal biography as well as an academic interest). However, in order to establish a reflexive context it is useful to think about the ways in which 'stepping' is understood in relation to fitness in the twenty-first century. It was also a coincidence that, on the day Figure 3.1 was taken I happened to be teaching about the sporting body and relationships of power that particular morning and had included photos of a modern step machine (Figure 3.2) as well as historical photos of prisoners being made to 'exercise' on a treadmill in a Victorian prison.

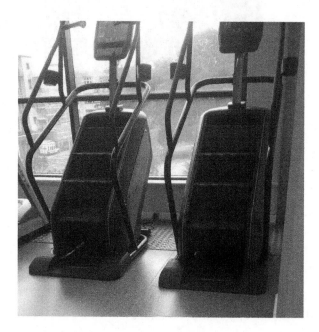

FIGURE 3.2 Step machines in a contemporary gym

The prisoners were engaging in a daily activity that was considered part of their punishment and also a means of gainfully occupying the men during the day. Apparently, in many cases the men could be made to endure the treadmills for hours on end. I used Figure 3.2 as a discussion point and compared it with the photos of the prisoners. It provided a useful way to highlight different forms of knowledge, and how the prisoners understood the treadmill in terms of a punishment and not as a positive healthy lifestyle activity in the way that a contemporary participant in a gym might understand the activity. There was an additional irony in that, although I showed the students the images and we had an opportunity to discuss the theoretical implications of how knowledge and power operate, I was unaware that the session my coach had planned for me in the afternoon involved a version of this activity in the form of repeated box steps. In this particular case, it involved a timed session where I had to do a series of step-ups on to a box while carrying a weighted barbell. It was probably no surprise that when I was doing the activity I thought about those prisoners and how they must have felt when they were made to do it. More specifically, I wondered how they were able to physically and mentally endure that activity. They were being forced to do it and had little choice in the matter. Nevertheless, they still had to develop strategies to be able to cope with the physical reality, especially if this was for several hours. Although the activity I performed only lasted for about 15 minutes and the intensity was different (and those men were not carrying additional weights on their back or climbing such high steps), it did still make me wonder how they managed to get through it. Obviously, a major difference between the context of a prison and a gym is that there is a greater element of choice about whether one takes part in a training session in a gym. Consequently, when I talk about enduring the sessions in my diary extracts I am still describing embodied experiences of pain and exhaustion which are often portrayed in a manner that is somewhat akin to a form of punishment. Although it is nothing like the context in which those men had to use the treadmill, there are still many questions that arise when trying to understand the context of a contemporary gym training session and the extent to which I have as much agency as I like to think. It might be the case that, if we think abstractly, the act of going to the gym or working out in the twenty-first century could be seen in terms of a form of punishment where the gym goer is subjugated, in as much as they are governed by a broader discourse of knowledge about fitness, health and how to act on the body, which effectively constitutes a form of prison. However, although there is leverage in this train of thought, it does not fully capture the broader embodied experience that entices me to go back for more.

Traditional sociology tends to adopt a 'top-down' approach to studying society through the way that it sets out to focus on the broader structures that shape and inform knowledge. And, although more qualitative forms of social research that explore individual experience have become more accepted within the discipline, it is, nevertheless, the influence of scientific discourses that expound objectivity and quantification that still remains dominant. Although I do not seek to identify or, indeed, reinforce the adoption of one over the other, it is difficult to avoid the historical foundations upon which sociology has been established. Consequently, the ideas presented in this book have been unapologetically developed through a subjective, qualitative approach in order to provide a form of response to the broader generalisations that are made about what health and physical activity are and should look like.

None the less, I do not seek to ignore the presence of broader social discourses. My intention of starting from an individual perspective is made by incorporating a sociological lens with the aim of avoiding the pitfall of many psychological accounts that focus only on the individual mind and often end up accepting the social body as given (and in turn position the individual as the problem in an unproblematic society). Consequently, my rationale is to remain mindful of these competing theories by adopting an embodied approach—one that, I believe, can accommodate the complexity of knowledge that is socially produced, constantly changing and also, ultimately, experienced in a range of contradictory ways by the individual. Within the context of health, physical activity and 'wellbeing', the need for an eclectic approach to understanding such ethereal and arbitrary concepts is even greater.

Healthy bodies

Shilling (2008) describes how social understandings of health and illness have changed over time. Specifically, he explains how, in western society, there has been a social transition from an initial understanding of a 'sick role', where being sick was understood in terms of the function it provided for society. Much of this understanding of sickness was generated through a relationship of sickness to production and labour—in other words, how an ill person could be accommodated during a period of ill-health and most effectively returned to the workplace. However, as Shilling describes:

> As the [20th] century came to a close, this emphasis led to a relative shift away from the institutional concern with sickness as a temporary deviation from the norm, towards a focus on

the imperative of maintaining health in order to conform to the values of an increasingly competitive and performative society.

(Shilling 2008, p. 106)

Shilling, drawing on Frank (1991), describes how during the course of the twentieth century there was a gradual move towards a 'health role'. This discourse of health differed from the sick role in that it was focused more upon 'the maximisation of people's productive capacities and the prevention of illness' (Shilling 2008, p. 106). Although the notion of an individual being productive was not new, this prioritisation of the prevention of illness, and regarding healthy bodies primarily in terms of the capacity to work and their productiveness in relation to the economy, can be seen to have been influential in the development of contemporary understandings of healthy lifestyles. A shift in social understanding of health emerged at the same time as more elaborate forms of surveillance both at a social level and at a personal level. These have been detailed in post-structural theory, in particular Foucault's descriptions of power, surveillance and sexuality (Foucault 1978, 1979, 1980) and subsequent theorising of biopower (Rose 2007). In addition, the emergence of broader political discourses that have eschewed neoliberal interpretations of consumerism (Phipps 2014) in maintaining the economy have also contributed to a more specific form of a material body. Subsequently, the health role that Shilling speaks of can be regarded as a significant aspect in the way that individuals understand and act upon their bodies.

These changes can be seen to compel individuals to be, at the very least, aware of their own responsibility in personal health maintenance—the emphasis here being that the physical body should be kept at its optimum state, in a way like a car that needs to be regularly serviced and maintained so that it holds its greatest value. According to Shilling, the health role creates a climate where individuals are urged to be at their fittest and the most adaptable they can be so that they can discharge their existing social roles and seek out new opportunities for engaging in productive activities. In order to do this, there is the knowledge that by investing in the health role one has an automatic right 'to a seemingly ever-expanding quantity of health related products and services' (Shilling 2008, p. 107). In other words, the knowledge about contemporary being is dominated by a discourse of economics, or western capitalism, that shapes the way an individual might think about the body as a material investment, which needs to be managed strategically and in similar way to how one should manage personal finances.

Although it is clear here that Shilling's arguments draw heavily from a traditional critical view of capitalism, it is also worth mentioning how other theorists, such as Pronger (2002), note how contemporary knowledge of the body not only promotes a way of perceiving the body in terms of a financial investment, but also creates a more disturbing form of (self-centred) body fascism. Technologies of fitness, and in particular those products of information and knowledge that are core to learning about how to get or how to become fit, become so entrenched in the everyday that they become unchallenged, and ultimately limit other expressions of being. I return to these debates later.

However, within the context of sport it is interesting to note how the notions of both the sick role and the health role contribute to understandings of the sporting and fit body. Although these are not necessarily complementary, they can be seen to operate in distinct parameters. In terms of the sick role, it might be argued that this still has resonance in the way that sickness is often understood alongside injury, and in this way considered as a temporary interruption before getting back into productive labour (or sporting activity). The health role, on the other hand, applies itself within sport much more in the context of the contribution that physical activity and sporting activity can make towards an individual's health and, consequently, their added productiveness within a broader work-based economy. Consequently, it is difficult to make firm claims that there has been a clear movement from one to another (not that Shilling is necessarily claiming this). However, there are obvious tensions between the two forms of thought and taking into account the contrasting contexts, such as a hospital or a gym, and these highlight the need for greater subjectivity. Bearing this in mind, as well as the themes that emerged in Chapter 2, it appears appropriate to further analyse the role of those involved in the process of 'fitness'. At the front line are personal trainers and the broader fitness industry. These are informed to varying degrees by health knowledge and government policies. Exploration of how they relate to each other and the context within which their roles have emerged reveals the complexity of relationships that are generated at the individual level (in terms of trainer and trained) and the broader social relationships (in terms of an industry that operates at both commercial and public health levels).

We are doing this for your own good

Often, when policy is framed in terms of an overall objective of obtaining greater wellbeing, the initial focus is not necessarily concerned with broader visions but rather single issues. For instance, much of recent government policy in England aimed at the welfare of children has been prompted more by focus upon a 'children as victims' discourse, fuelled by high-profile cases of apparent failings in Children's Services to protect vulnerable children (Powell & Wellard 2008). Using the example of children's wellbeing, recent policy in England affecting children (such as Every Child Matters—Department for Education and Skills 2004; and The Children's Plan—Department for Children, Schools and Families 2007) has consequently adopted measures that, intentionally or not, construct children as potentially at risk from a range of threats. On the one hand, this interpretation of children's wellbeing can be viewed as a positive step towards protecting children, whereas, on the other, it can equally be seen to restrict opportunities for children to experience and learn about the wider world on their own terms (Furedi 2008, Lester & Russell 2008).

The example of the conflicting messages about what is 'good' for children reveals how these have a direct impact on the ways in which not only children, but also adults, can experience their bodies and explore spaces. For instance, examples in sport can be seen in other social categories considered 'at risk', such as women runners (Clark 2013), disabled athletes (Brighton 2014), the older athlete (Baker et al. 2010, Humberstone 2010). Within the specific context of sport and physical activity, messages about the positive effects are generally described in relation to physical health and the prevention of disease in later life (Sallis & Owen 1999). Research has also tended to concentrate on the relationship of the benefits of physical activity, sport and play to cognitive and academic development, mental health, crime reduction, and reduction of truancy and disaffection (Bailey 2005). The focus on the role of physical activity, sport and play has emerged from a general belief that the health and wellbeing of the population should be a national concern, in a way that presents young people as well as adults of being 'at risk' of not undertaking enough physical activity. Consequently, in the quest to address the perceived imbalances within social wellbeing, there has been much focus on bodies and minds, particularly in relation to perceived healthy lifestyle behaviours. For example, in the UK there have been several major national interventions, such as the Change4Life programme, which have, through substantial government investment, attempted to promote, and change attitudes to health and physical activity.[1]

Although it is reasonable to suggest that the underlying agenda for any international organisation concerned with the interests of children and adults should be related to addressing the problems of global poverty, in wealthier 'western' countries, or as Connell (2007) calls it 'the Metropole', there has been more focus on wellbeing expressed in terms of 'health' and potential risk of obesity (Gard & Wright 2005). Physical activity, sport and play have therefore become even more appealing to policy-makers and educationalists seeking explanations for perceived 'risky' behaviours, such as sedentary lifestyles in children and adults. Indeed, there has been much interest in childhood behaviour and possible connections between poor nutrition and inactivity with cognitive development (Heller et al. 2011, Nyaradi et al. 2013), which is considered a key aspect of health-related wellbeing. Consequently, wellbeing and health have been defined as important 'products' of children's physical activity, sport and play, thus providing the basis for their inclusion in educational curricula and out-of-school programmes and provision (Bailey et al. 2009). In their concerns to address the perceived 'problems' of children's health, policy-makers have invariably targeted schools as a prime site for introducing mechanisms to address them. However, as Gard (2011) points out:

> From the public health perspective, schools are simply assumed to represent new target populations, little different from any other, without any sense that unique challenges might exist or that new methods might be called for.
>
> *(Gard 2011, p. 404)*

Staying with the example of children, where public health policies are generated with well-intentioned motives related to protecting the interests of children, an unintended (or in some cases intended) consequence is that continued focus on specific outcomes (such as tackling obesity or increasing physical activity levels) has side-lined many other equally important aspects of a young person's development, such as creativity and personal enjoyment (Gard 2006, Wellard 2013). As a result, there is continued lack of recognition of the multifaceted interplay of the physical, social and psychological ways in which individuals develop an orientation towards their own embodied identity, and subsequently whether they interpret health-related activities as personally meaningful.

Much of the debate above can be seen to be fuelled by lack of clarity over what wellbeing actually means. Although some consider the concept less problematic and, indeed, approach it in terms of a more measureable 'object', which invariably incorporates economic determinants (Tennant et al. 2007, Dolan & Metcalfe 2012), it is more likely that pursuit of a uniform definition is always going to be fraught with tensions (Evans et al. 2004, Vernon, 2008, Ahmed 2010). However, although I suggest that attempting to define wellbeing is always going to be problematic, it is important to look briefly at why it is problematic in the first place. If we think of wellbeing in philosophical terms, we are drawn into the ontological assessment of an individual state of being. In this case, wellbeing is often contemplated in terms of individual pleasure and states of happiness. Vernon (2008) attempts to look at the meaning beyond the actual or intrinsic feeling of pleasure and suggests that, although wellbeing derives from happiness it is less subjective. In a similar manner to the contemplation of happiness, most of the questions relating to it are framed in terms of 'how do we achieve it'. As Vernon suggests, part of the modern-day obsession with finding happiness is influenced heavily by consumerist discourses where 'keeping up with the Joneses' is something that in itself becomes pleasurable, and this fuels a market place of easy, pleasurable luxuries which invariably (and ironically) creates unhappiness (Vernon 2008, p. 23).

The consumerist discourses that Vernon mentions have become so ingrained in our everyday thinking that they ultimately generate a greater perception that consumer choice is a right in itself. As early as the latter stages of the twentieth century Graham (1995) noted how the business model of 'consumer choice' was being applied to American schools. In doing so, this approach opened up debate about the notion of 'listening' to student voices in the context of them being customers. The idea of considering a student in terms of a 'happy' customer created uneasy tensions with existing philosophies within education and healthcare, where the decisions practitioners were making were ultimately believed to be 'for the good' of their students or patients. Graham's ideas were generated during a time when there was much work produced on the effects of consumer lifestyles (e.g. Bourdieu 1986, Tomlinson 1990, Featherstone 1991, Urry 1995), where the notion that individual happiness or wellbeing has been shaped through a quest to constantly keep up with others reflected a contemporary formulation of what is required to achieve a perceived ideal state of being. It is interesting, however, to consider the role of the personal trainer within these discussions because the notion of relationships between a teacher and student or doctor and patient have been developed over time, whereas the personal trainer is a relatively new occupation. In this role, the personal trainer has been created very much 'within' a business model in which the relationship is with a client. What is interesting is that, with the emergence of the personal trainer and subsidiary health advisors, there appears to be a move towards emulating the professional and social standing of teachers and doctors in order to make the role much more marketable. (I explore this further later in this chapter.) Nevertheless, these ideas very much necessitate a sociocultural perspective of how our relationships with others affect perceived states of happiness or wellbeing.

Relationships of power

It is reasonable to assert that there are complicated relationships of power that affect the way that individuals can interact with others and, indeed, 'exist'. These operate through forms of knowledge, economic power, and formal and informal structures that contribute to the management of bodies and society (Shilling 1993). However, rather than attempt to make claims that there are dominant forms of power, available to certain groups, which are consciously oppressing other groups, it is more appropriate to explore the forms of power that are operating (or prevailing) in order to understand how they are being acted upon or reacted to. To this extent, a Foucauldian interpretation of discourses of power provides an extremely relevant approach to investigate sport and physical cultures (Andrews 1993, Smith Maguire 2002). By adopting this approach, it is suggested that, rather than attempting to eliminate oppressive power, it should be considered as omnipresent in every interaction and action (Andrews 1993) and, instead of omitting power altogether, it is necessary to investigate how it is used within physical activity, exercise and sport (Markula 2003).

When Foucault refers to power he is not referring to a 'substance', but instead he discusses power as a particular form of relationship between people. The distinctive aspect of power is that some individuals can shape the actions of others, but not necessarily in a coercive manner. Through ever-present inequalities, power relationships are always provoking positions of power, although these positions are specific in each location and changeable. Power is omnipresent. In addition, power is always coupled with resistance, which is not external to power relationships. In a similar way to power relationships, however, resistance is not regular; it is moveable and changeable within the complex network of power relationships (Foucault 1978). Put in another way, a relationship of power is not an act on another individual but rather an action on another action (Foucault 1978, 1979). For power relationships to exist, the 'other' has to be deemed as an individual who acts, and a number of reactions, results and responses must be possible when faced with this power relationship. Power relationships are entrenched within a whole society and social structures, and are never stable or finite (Foucault 1980, 1985).

Consequently, despite the notion that dominant groups, governments and social institutions possess power, Foucault (1978) argues that they symbolise only power that can be ended (Markula & Pringle 2006). Foucault refused to understand power as something that was owned by some, and used to control those with no power (Andrews 1993, Smith Maguire 2002). He explained that these dominant groups do not simply inherit their dominant positions because of the power they possess, but instead they gain their dominance because of the changeable working and strategic use of 'discourses' (Pringle & Markula 2005). It takes the analysis of history and power to understand these workings and gain the opportunity to change them (Markula & Pringle 2006). The continued utility of applying Foucault's genealogical approach to relationships of power is neatly summarised by Phipps (2014), when she describes the reason for her use of this approach in her study of contemporary feminism and body politics was fuelled by a concern with the following:

> How the discussions themselves are constructed: the concepts and rhetorics or 'regimes of truth' (Foucault 1980: 131) deployed, the political allegiances being made, and their contextual conditions of possibility.
>
> *(Phipps 2014, p. 4)*

Although I do not propose to present, in this chapter, a genealogy of power within the context of either fitness-related pursuits or personal training, I am, nevertheless, seeking to understand the will to know the truth operating in relation to 'wellbeing'. In doing so, it is worth asking the three central questions that Foucault (1985) considered crucial in the process of forming enunciative modalities. These relate to identifying who is speaking (what institutions are speaking), the site of the discourse and who is the listener (Foucault 1985, p. 50). Posing these questions reveals the relationships of power that are 'in play' before and during a social situation such as personal training or the social space of a gym. Thus we might apply these questions to help us understand the knowledge structures at large that are shaping perceptions of wellbeing or what a healthy body should 'look like'. In this case, the institutions that are speaking are commercial industries, government (health) organisations, and trainers who are formulating how fitness can be developed, presented and sold. Each 'group' can be seen to have a broad 'shared' vision for the enhanced wellbeing of their 'clients'. They are similarly linked through contemporary discourses of public policy, informed by a mix of medical and economic theory, and generated through scientific and western capitalist discourses. However, at the same time, each could be seen to have different interpretations of what wellbeing is as well as contrasting agendas and ideas for how such a vision can be translated into practice.

One way to consider these complex relationships can be seen in Figure 3.3. This is provided as a simple illustration of some of the often competing forms of power that are operating at any one time and highlights the competing and conflicting interpretations of a concept that at face value is 'shared' (Figure 3.3).

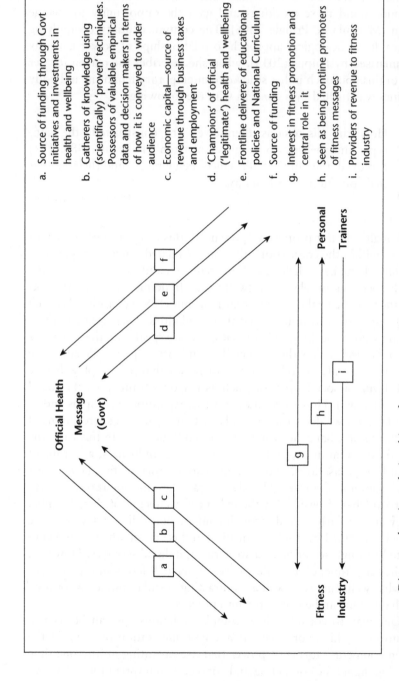

a. Source of funding through Govt initiatives and investments in health and wellbeing

b. Gatherers of knowledge using (scientifically) 'proven' techniques. Possessors of valuable empirical data and decision makers in terms of how it is conveyed to wider audience

c. Economic capital—source of revenue through business taxes and employment

d. 'Champions' of official ('legitimate') health and wellbeing

e. Frontline deliverer of educational policies and National Curriculum

f. Source of funding

g. Interest in fitness promotion and central role in it

h. Seen as being frontline promoters of fitness messages

i. Providers of revenue to fitness industry

FIGURE 3.3 Diagram showing relationships of power operating across government, fitness industries and personal trainers

The relationships that operate across these groups (as well as many others) are dynamic and constantly shifting. There are, however, forms of power that can be seen to be more beneficial to one group than another. These are indicated by the direction of the arrowheads in Figure 3.3.

In critical sociology, debates about the role of the state in everyday life are abundant. For instance, Habermas's (1989) description of the private and public sphere has been interpreted in various forms. However, as Bennett (2006) suggests, the advantages of superimposing a Foucauldian perspective on the historical processes that Habermas is concerned with are in how it provides a way of recognising and, subsequently, thinking about the various forms of relationships at play and the ways in which 'cultural resources are organized to act on the social in different ways in accordance with shifting governmental conceptions and priorities' (Bennett 2006, p. 99).

Although questions about the dynamics of the 'state' are not the focus of this book, I remain mindful of the influence that wider debate has had on the way in which I explore health and wellbeing. It is useful to consider, as Bennett (2006, p. 87) does, Hunter's (1994) notion of 'secular holiness', which is itself a critique of the perceived position of the critical intellectual as detached from the bureaucrat. Consequently, the relationships of power illustrated in Figure 3.3 are intended to highlight the interconnectedness rather than disconnectedness of the institutions operating within these discourses of power. At the same time, my attempts to identify some of these power relationships assist in my effort to remain reflexive in the way that I approach my thinking— not only in terms of the central questions posed throughout the book but also as a mechanism to remain alert to what might be considered my fluctuating allegiances with the various groups.

I continue by exploring the forms of power that might be seen to ultimately shape the way in which each of the groups 'sees' the role of physical activity promotion.

Personal trainers

In the introduction I described how I had previously developed what might be considered a slight distrust of personal trainers in terms of how I was not always convinced about their broader 'body knowledge'. Nevertheless, the emergence of their role in recent years as that of health advisors is interesting from a sociological perspective, in terms of its uneasy relationship between established public and private sector roles, such as the medical doctor and the business entrepreneur.

Consequently, the themes that emerged during my training and identified in Chapter 2 highlight the complex relationships of trust informed by wider social knowledge, as well as the personal dynamics of a one-to-one encounter. In my case, my initial reservations about personal trainers has been informed by my exposure to knowledge about health and fitness as well as the health role that Shilling describes. Although the context of my relationship with a personal trainer is subjective in that my personal history has been influenced by a range of factors (such as academic background, sporting ability, gender, age and so on), like anyone else entering into a social encounter, I go through a process of assessing my own presumptions and weigh these up with the subsequent embodied experience of the activity. In this way, the varying expressions of trust that are operating in my experiences while training with coach JP, although not necessarily exactly the same, are, nevertheless, comparable to others entering into a period of physical training (whether, for instance, through a GP referral or in an attempt to lose weight). These relationships are not governed by forms of straightforward dominance where one individual has power over another, but are much more complex and dynamic. A session with a personal trainer provides a good example, precisely because it highlights the forms of power that are not only operating between the participants but also influenced by a range of competing social discourses generated about the body, health, fitness, age, ability, consumer culture and so much more.

In Chapter 2 I described in the diary entries how I enjoyed learning about the capabilities of my body and being guided in routines and exercises that I had subconsciously (or probably consciously) avoided when training on my own. At the same time, I enjoyed the subtle forms of power relationships that I mention above, where I was the one that had to follow the lead and be told what to do, in the same way that I enjoy having opportunities to listen to a lecture rather than presenting one. The sessions, therefore, embraced a range of physical and social experiences that allowed me to feel comfortable putting myself 'in the hands' of the trainer. The important point here is that, in these circumstances, and within this context, I am complicit in this relationship of power and allow myself to be at times subservient, because I recognise that I have something to gain from this exchange. I am, however, aware of the subjectivity in these accounts of my experiences and I am sure this is not always the case in the relationships that are forged within the context of many other gym spaces and settings where those engaging are entering with different expectations and motivations and where other factors might be more significant (such as losing weight, altering outward physical appearance or, from the perspective of the personal trainer, generating income from 'clients').

What is important is the way that I have developed preconceptions about specific 'roles' within society. The coach, teacher and doctor are understood in terms of my awareness of the social prestige that is conferred upon these identities, and the knowledge that there are required 'professional' qualifications to reassure the public that those claiming these titles have done so after going through a rigorous form of training and gaining nationally recognised qualifications. Smith Maguire (2008) explores the role of professionalism within the context of personal training. She sees this as a discursive construction that is particularly revealing because of the tensions between that of providing a professional, service-based activity while also adopting more entrepreneurial aspects of selling a specific service. According to Smith Maguire, personal training is interesting in that personal trainers are paid to design and facilitate personal fitness programmes on a one-to-one basis. It is their position within a consumerist discourse, however, that places them almost as intermediaries between paying clients and broader larger fitness and exercise industry. She notes:

> In the experiences of fitness that they shape and the images of fitness that they embody, personal trainers help to educate consumers in a particular view of the body as a vehicle of self-expression and a focal point for consumption.
>
> *(Smith Maguire 2008, p. 212)*

For Smith Maguire, in general, social cultural research on fitness and aerobics has tended to focus on the participants rather than the practitioners. This is an important point and may help to explain why understandings of personal trainer/client relationships are more often than not described in terms of a binary factor where the personal trainer 'does' things 'to' or 'for' a client. Although this is relevant, personal trainers can also be considered participants in as much as they have invested the same values and ethos and discursive constructs that they are promoting. Motivations such as these might contrast with the notion of an entrepreneur who is interested in making profit rather than necessarily participating in or with the product that he or she promotes and sells. It could be claimed that, to a greater degree than a traditional teacher, personal trainers need to be seen to engage and practise what they preach. It is the case that much of the knowledge they display is initially presented through a body that has been perfected and is identifiable as representing 'fitness'. In contrast, school teachers do not necessarily need to 'demonstrate' their authenticity in such obvious ways because the status of 'teacher' brings with it understanding of prior learning and legitimate qualifications. However, it is noticeable, in more recent years, that there has been a concerted shift within the fitness industry to establish training routes and standard qualifications.[2]

Through analysis of personal training texts, Smith Maguire incorporates Bourdieu's (1984) theory of distinction and in particular the notion of cultural intermediaries who present and re-present as institutions providing symbolic goods and services.

Although Smith Maguire's focus is on how more traditional discursive structures relate to forms of professionalisation that influence the way that personal training has been developed, an important point that she raises relates to the ways in which the industry of personal training has been characterised by normative codes 'that place service before self-interest and justify the prestige of the profession by reference to a greater social cause' (Smith Maguire 2008, p. 217). The point here is that personal training tries to sell itself in terms of a public service. As such, its selling point is related to the idea that it is providing something of benefit to the public and, in doing so, attempts to align itself with other public services located within health.

Although Smith Maguire does not refer to him in her paper, Pronger's (2002) discussion of the technologies of fitness provides an important and more detailed discussion of the discursive constructs of the fitness industry. In particular, he identifies specific 'texts' that construct knowledge about fitness and individual bodies in contemporary western society. Pronger describes this as an 'intertextual ensemble' which includes five key fields or elements (see the section in this chapter entitled *Fitness industry*).

Personal trainers, as central representatives of this knowledge, are pivotal to the dissemination of this intertextual ensemble. It might also be suggested that they are in far less of a position to challenge or provide any level of academic 'resistance' because it is not in their interests to do so or included in their training as a form of critical reflection (although this may not necessarily be the case in current medical and teacher training). Consequently, the identity of the personal trainer is complex precisely because it operates through a range of discourses relating to a healthy body and contemporary formulations of an attractive, desirable body, as well as aspiring to be a public health promoter and entrepreneur.

Government agencies

The role of government agencies is increasingly seen in terms of the way that they can 'manage' social and political problems and convert them into market terms. According to Phipps (2014, p. 11):

> through channels such as government policy, advertising and popular culture, neoliberalism has become a normative framework, based on the idea of citizens as rational and self-interested economic actors with agency and control over their lives.

Thus, for example, obesity is interpreted within the neoliberal context that Phipps (2014) describes as an issue of individual responsibility and lifestyle choice rather than related to broader social determinants such as inequality and class (Evans, Davies and Wright 2004). By recognising the influence of contemporary social discourses on the way that knowledge is generated allows us to penetrate deeper into the relative quagmire that is wellbeing. For instance, Ereaut and Whiting's (2008) research into the ways in which wellbeing is defined and interpreted within an English government department reveals the contrasting way in which it is understood. In their research, they attempted to offer ways in which it can (or should) be understood in order to maintain consistency. Their main conclusion was that, in order to make sense of the way that wellbeing is understood and, subsequently, operates, is by acknowledging that it is foremost a social construct.

> There are no uncontested biological, spiritual, social, economic or any other kind of markers for wellbeing. The meaning of wellbeing is not fixed—it cannot be. It is a primary cultural judgement; just like 'what makes a good life?' it is the stuff of fundamental philosophical debate. What it means at any one time depends on the weight given at that time to different philosophical traditions, world views and systems of knowledge.
>
> *(Ereaut & Whiting 2008, p. 9)*

In their study, the researchers found that for many of the respondents 'wellbeing' was not necessarily a familiar term and it was difficult to apply the concept in a context that readily appealed to personal sentiments. In most cases, when pressed, the respondents offered interpretations that related to health and access to basic provisions considered necessary for a reasonable standard of living, such as food, water and housing. To an extent, they were applying similar descriptions to indicators of poverty, which itself has constantly been reassessed (Dornan & Veit-Wilson 2004, Alcock 2006). However, a central issue that helps unified thinking about standards of living is its relationship to economics. In the case of wellbeing, Ereaut and Whiting (2008) found that what could be considered an apparently central issue in a government department's strategy was not uniformly understood. Much of this ambiguity related to the age-old debates of theory and practice. Whereas an issue such as poverty, although open to theoretical debate as a concept, can be addressed in terms of economic measures to 'reduce' levels and increase overall standards of living, in the case of wellbeing the philosophical visions do not sit so easily with the operational requirements, particularly in the way in which it can be measured. Although it may be considered as a useful template, according to Ereaut and Whiting (2008, p. 19): 'the operationalised definition will never fully represent the broad ambition. It cannot, in that it does not fully meet wider societal understanding of wellbeing, and perhaps was never intended to'.

Nevertheless, within the context of a government agency, there is little time (or possibly little enthusiasm) for philosophical debates about the complexities of defining wellbeing. In some of the programmes that I have been involved with in the past, wellbeing was seen as unproblematic by the government agencies responsible for the intervention (and funding) in that it was considered an achievable outcome. For example, in a recent initiative aiming to get young people more active and funded by central government in England, the perception was that, through the introduction of a programme that could develop a child's physical literacy, it was considered reasonable to assume that the overarching intervention would be providing opportunities to promote individual responsibility and healthy lifestyle choices. However, the initial 'thinking' behind a concept such as physical literacy could be seen to be influenced by previous thinking about the role of sport and physical education (PE) in society. In this case, according to the agency involved physical literacy was measurable as it:

> helps primary school children's development as competent, confident and healthy movers at an early stage. It builds their motivation, confidence, physical competence and understanding of movement, providing them with better grounds to sustain their lifelong participation in physical activity.
>
> *(Youth Sport Trust 2013)*

Physical literacy was considered an outcome that would emerge 'within' PE and sport provision, particularly in the teaching of core movement skills. However, it could be argued that the historical formulation of PE in the UK that Kirk (1992) outlines plays a significant part in the way that the concept is approached. The interpretation of physical literacy in England could be seen to be in contrast to other interpretations and variations on the theme, such as 'health literacy' (Kilgour et al. 2013), 'sport literacy' (Pill 2010) and 'movement literacy' (Kentel & Dobson 2007). So, although physical literacy has been embraced as a concept (at an international level) to engage people in a form of embodied consciousness, where the benefits of increased activity can be internalised positively, the actual interpretation and practice varied from country to country. For example, across the border from England, Wales was rolling out a similar national strategy at the same time. However, their approach adopted a much broader understanding in which physical literacy could develop in all aspects of the curriculum and not just sport and physical education:

> The Vision for Sport in Wales is that 'Every child and young person is provided with the skills and confidence from an early age to be physically literate through high quality, engaging experiences'.
> *(Sport Wales 2010, p. 31)*

In this case, the programme introduced by Sport Wales was a whole school intervention which focused on numeracy and literacy as an outcome that could be addressed through physical literacy via PE and school sport. Consequently, the perception and interpretation of physical literacy was (and is) being very much shaped by the socio-political and historical 'location' of the government agency tasked with implementing the intervention.

Fitness industry

Fitness is big business. According to the 2017 State of UK fitness industry report (see www.leisuredb.com/blog/2017/5/5/2017-state-of-the-uk-fitness-industry-report-out-now), 9.7 million people were members of a gym, equating to one in seven of the overall UK population. For many, engaging in gyms and recreational leisure is a form of 'serious leisure' (Stebbins 2006). Although the training of the physical body and engagement in sporting activities have an established presence in cultural history, albeit with varying interpretations and implementation at different historical stages, the notion of a fitness 'industry' is a relatively new phenomenon. The industry that is described today can be seen to emerge in its current form during the late twentieth century (Chaline 2015) and is heavily influenced by consumption practices, to the extent that gym membership now appears compulsory in order to become a legitimate member of late modern, neo-liberal, capitalist society (e.g. Sassetelli 2015).

The increase in the popularity of fitness-related pursuits provides further support for Shilling's (2008) claims about the shift in thinking about health as well as a body that can be perfected. The notion of a perfectible body has been explored extensively in post-structuralist theory (Low & Malacrida 2008), but, in the case of fitness, Pronger's (2002) use of the work of Foucault in illuminating a form of body fascism, in which the ubiquity of the perfect body creates a panoptic effect as individuals watch over themselves for any deviations from these norms, provides a compelling argument. For him, using a gym and committing to a 'body project' are therefore not exclusively an expression of individual agency, but policed through the adherence to, or docility towards, dominant cultural discourses (Foucault 1979). These discourses of knowledge or 'technologies of fitness' (Pronger 2002, p. 123) are generated through what he describes as 'five texts':

1. government fitness initiatives, policies and position statements on health such as recommended PA levels;
2. articles, textbooks and educational resource materials (such as sports science);
3. popular magazines, books and videos on fitness and health;
4. exercise prescriptions, health appraisals, sport and fitness equipment, the tools used to monitor, control and increase fitness levels; and
5. popular media representations of the 'fit' body.

The focus on discourse is valuable in illuminating how understanding of the gym, or participating in a gym, has been socially constructed. However, it could be argued that such accounts are discursively essentialist and fall short in representing the fleshiness of embodied experience. Indeed, as Pronger acknowledged, often it is the case that the more embodied aspects of physical activity are overlooked. For instance, in the case of PE practices, subjective aspects such as pleasure or desire are not featured in any discussions on how young people could be active, 'except negatively where physical education is constructed as strategic in the control of desire (the desire to indulge in delicious, fattening foods, for example)' (Pronger 2002, p. 8). At the time of writing this, Pronger suggested that a positive sense of the body's pleasure and desire could make a positive contribution to developing a greater understanding of the body.

Embodied approaches: filling in the gaps

Although the contribution of post-structuralism to our understanding of knowledge is obviously significant, discussion about discourse is always going to be abstract and, although the notion of the body as a focus of power relationships has been established, there is still room for further discussion relating to embodied experience. The discussion above has been very much about knowledge and discourses of fitness. The knowledge that is available to me has influenced the way that I am able to approach and take part in sport and physical activity. However, to an extent, identifying the prevailing knowledge structures is a starting point in my quest to understand in more depth what it is about physical activity that maintains my desire to engage, and keep engaging. I mention this because it is apparent that many other people do not engage in physical activity to the same extent. So, although the discourses of knowledge, influenced by scientific evidence and government policy, emphatically endorse the benefits of an active lifestyle, it is still apparent that a significant proportion of the population does not act upon this (Sport England 2017).

I have no intention of making this book into some form of health promotion pamphlet. Indeed, as it will become clearer in subsequent chapters, there are many aspects of my (and others) engagement in physical activity that might be considered not necessarily conducive to overall physical health or wellbeing. The point being made is that the generalised messages about healthy, physical activity behaviours, informed as they are through objective, evidence-based research, do not accommodate enough recognition (if any) of the subjective and experiential factors that play such a significant part in any form of engagement in social and physical activities.

Consequently, although I can put hands up and say that I love 'doing' sport and physical activity, there are still times when I do not want to engage as enthusiastically, or even at all. Various factors influence the way that I choose to engage or not, such as the time of day, the weather, how I am feeling (physically and mentally) after a hard day's work, whether I feel like being with other people and so on. Nevertheless, when I am in the right frame of mind and my body feels up to it (which is more often, than not), I enjoy the experience in many ways (see Wellard 2013). However, although I am an advocate of the 'joys' of taking part in physical activities, I remain suspicious about the many (sometimes sanctimonious) promoters of health-related physical fitness who appear to believe physical activity is an unproblematic direct line to wellbeing and can be readily incorporated into everyday routines, regardless of the individual's circumstances.

Much of this suspicion about many of those who preach the (unproblematic) benefits of fitness is that they fail to acknowledge how an individual creates corporeal understanding of their own body and the significance that this plays in developing understanding of their own and others' physical identities. For instance, when thinking about embodied experiences within the gym, I suggest that an embodied approach helps assist in developing a theoretical position that acknowledges the role of the body in shaping external practices—more specifically, a form of embodied understanding that incorporates a social constructionist approach, but also includes the lived, feeling body within social processes (Wellard 2013).

The embodied approach that I have developed draws on Connell's (1995) circuit of body-reflexive practices as a starting point for understanding how social and cultural factors entwine with individual bodily experiences. Body-reflexive practices, for Connell, are formed through a circuit of bodily interactions and experiences via socially constructed understandings of the body, which lead to new bodily interactions. She argues that the corporeality of the body needs to be accounted for within social theory, and 'through body-reflexive practices, bodies are addressed by social process and drawn into history, without ceasing to be bodies . . . they do not turn into symbols, signs or positions in discourse' (Connell 2005, p. 64). Connell developed this approach as a way of exploring how the gendered body had (has) been constructed through a masculine lens. Attributing the notion of a circuit of body-reflexive pleasures enables the possibility of incorporating an embodied approach to other practices, such as physical activity.

I initially applied Connell's concept so that I could understand the notion of a circuit of body-reflexive pleasures (Wellard 2013), located in the context of the body, and sport and physical activities. Within this context, I was attempting to explore the complex range of factors that contribute towards an individual's experiences of pleasure (or not) when engaging in physical activities. Here, the intention was to highlight that, to understand a person's experience of sport, greater acknowledgement needs to be made of the social, psychological and physiological processes that occur at any situation, and how each may influence the experience at varying levels. In this case, a central part of this circuit was considered to be pleasure where the interconnected factors related to engaging in a physical activity determine an individual's experience, and these have varying degrees of influence on an experience. I was, subsequently, able to make further claims that different 'times' and 'spaces' impact on how a certain activity is experienced as fun. Considering space enables the opportunity to approach space and place as more fluid and, by doing so, challenge the often immobile developments of this concept (Figure 3.4).

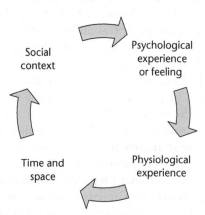

FIGURE 3.4 Circuit of body-reflexive pleasure (Wellard 2013)

The acknowledgement of spatial and temporal factors within the circuit was incorporated so that I could develop a deeper understanding of how pleasure is more than an insignificant or 'one-off' moment of self-gratification. Pleasure can be considered as a process in terms of how an experience can *become* pleasurable as well as a moment. Consequently, this circuit describes pleasure as a continuously moving process, and incorporates the inclusion of anticipation, experience and reflection.

An individual's orientation towards thinking about pain and pleasure has often been contextualised as a necessary and essential element in performance progress. Thinking about the body in this way has filtered into amateur sports and broader health and fitness industries. An example of this is the motivational aspects used within fitness training, where the mantras of 'no pain, no gain' and 'feel the burn' are accepted (and expected) practice. Therefore, a more complicated relationship between pleasure and pain is present due to physical pain being rearticulated by an individual, so the experience can be re-evaluated in a more pleasurable and positive way. The social context of how an activity (such as performed in a gym) can be regulated in different social spaces highlights the various ways in which an individual's embodiedness is experienced, particularly within sport and physical activity contexts.

As a result, adopting an embodied approach helps us incorporate the discourses of knowledge that create an orientation to a particular activity, but allows us to move beyond the abstract discussions and attempt to include the physical experience, the spatial context and the temporal aspects. Thus, the figures of the prisoners and myself engaging in physical activity can be interpreted through the discourses of knowledge surrounding punishment, health and physical activity—relating to specific historical periods. However, an embodied approach helps us dig a little bit deeper and recognise the various ways in which the individual internalises 'outside' forms of knowledge and acts on them. However, although the initial assessment of the prisoners might take into account a scenario in which the men are being made to do the exercises because of the way that the role of the prison has been interpreted at that particular socio-historic moment, it does not fully accommodate the experience of the men taking part. We might assume that the men are being forced to do the activity, but this does not necessarily mean that the activity was experienced and understood as a punishment, or automatically unenjoyable. If the treadmill were the only opportunity for physical activity, it could be reasonable to suggest that some prisoners might have been more positive about the opportunity to engage in physical exercise and be away from the confines of their cell and their cellmates. Similarly, many may look at the activity that I was performing and think about it as being something that they would not willingly want to do.

Health and fitness knowledge

Although I identified three 'key players' in the production of health and fitness knowledge, it is worth mentioning the role of academics. Although my methodological approach is to remain constantly aware that I am a social actor residing within the field that I am attempting to understand, as an academic I am also not immune to other forms of knowledge that influence academia, such as an audit culture (Sparkes 2007) and the complex relationships of power operating at large, governed by performance indicators (Ball 2004). My 'position' as an academic, as well as occasionally a researcher commissioned to explore the impact of public funded programmes (such as the one mentioned above), also creates many tensions. It is often the case that in large-scale projects such as these the researchers involved have different academic 'histories' shaped by what might be considered conflicting theoretical approaches. The academics involved in many of the projects that I have been involved in had backgrounds in sociology, physiology, politics, policy and psychology. Nevertheless, as academic researchers we did have strategies in place to help us attempt to overcome such potential conflicts (compared with the other groups). For instance, in the physical literacy programme mentioned earlier, the research team attempted to establish a 'baseline' understanding of physical literacy, guided by the concept developed by Whitehead (2010). Here, physically, literacy is described as 'the motivation, confidence, physical competence, knowledge and understanding to maintain physical activity throughout the lifecourse' (Whitehead 2010).

Although this definition might have been incorporated in the overarching mission statement for the intervention, I cannot be certain that the government agency coordinating the intervention and the schools taking part would necessarily be interpreting the theoretical 'position' in the way in which the academics did. Indeed, I could not be certain that the other academics involved in the research project shared my interpretation, which was one that acknowledges the philosophical origins of a concept derived through influences from existentialism, phenomenology and embodiment (Whitehead 2010, Wellard 2013). Nevertheless, it also meant that the research team was operating within a competing knowledge structure in which physical literacy is understood as a 'monist' concept with the mind and body not seen as separate. Consequently, we were, at once, separating ourselves from the established discourse operating within contemporary social thinking, where the two are generally considered as separate and social structures have been developed in ways that accommodate this distinction (Evans et al. 2004). However, a monist approach to understanding physical literacy appealed to our academic sensibilities as well as the general 'vision' that we had established in creating a university-based research centre.

Laying one's 'cards on the table' does not necessarily mean that one will always be in direct opposition to those who are involved in research, whether or not they are stakeholders or the specific focus of the research. Indeed, it could equally be claimed that there are many connections that are revealed in the process of adopting such a reflexive stance. Nevertheless, the discussion in this chapter highlights the tensions between the rhetoric of individual expression and the restraints of performative agendas operating through government policy and broader social and cultural imperatives.

Although this chapter has only touched on the outer layers of a range of complex and competing issues, the intention was to do just that because there is the underlying recognition of the greater depth lurking beneath. However, the point made here is that there is a broader context to my participation in this training programme, informed by knowledge generated historically in often contrasting sites.

These all inform the way that I experience such an activity and, although these experiences are subjective at the individual level, they provide the opportunity to reflect on and contemplate not only processes that occur in physical activity participation, but also broader debates about being.

In the following chapters, I draw on themes that became more significant in my continued participation in the training.

Notes

1 Change4Life is a flagship programme of Public Health England for preventing childhood obesity. The programme aims through a series of public interventions to improve health behaviours, such as poor diet and lack of physical activity, which can lead to obesity, particularly in children.

2 For instance, in the UK, basic requirements for employment as a personal trainer are managed through industry-recognised qualifications administered through the Register for Exercise Professionals (REPS).

4

WHAT PAIN?

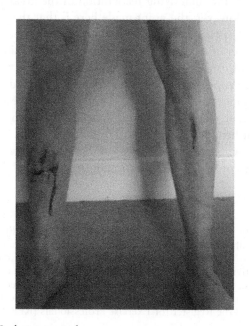

FIGURE 4.1 Workout wounds

Suffering for my art

I was only joking with a colleague the other day that the research I'm doing is like the French artist ORLAN, who uses her body as the object of her art. By putting herself under the knife and undergoing plastic surgery she says that her body becomes the object of her art. I suppose it's stretching the point just a little bit but it is interesting to think about the research process and the extent to which embodied researchers place their bodies as a central focus for their research so that they can attempt to understand how they respond physically and emotionally to lived experience.

Although this was meant to be a joke at the time, there are some comparisons that I can make to the notion of using my body as an experiment and rather than it being an artistic experiment it is still the focus of a sociological experiment. Indeed, the whole point of doing this research and going through the process of experiencing this training programme has been for me to experience all the embodied aspects so that I can reflect upon them with a sociological imagination. I'm not meaning to sound really grand (and I can hear myself flinching at the possible pompousness of these words) but experiencing those lived moments is really important. Although the primary intention of embodied research is to bridge the gap between theory and practice, there is, nevertheless, the constant fear that only focusing on theory can sometimes take over and miss vital elements of lived practice. In particular, what I'm trying to say is that it can be sometimes easy for academics to remain detached from what they are studying and then attempt to make assumptions about what an experience might look like, feel like and 'be' like.

So then, what has made me think about all of this? Because today in the session I managed to fall arse over head during the start of the planned WoD [workout of the day] and the embodied experience threw up quite a few unexpected thoughts (and feelings, both physical and emotional) that I may not have fully grasped if I had tried to imagine the scenario. It's later in the day now and I'm sitting on the sofa with my feet up, feeling sore and a little bit sorry for myself. However, I wasn't going to let what happened pass by without milking it for all of its (embodied) theoretical possibilities. It's true, that while I was sitting on the floor nursing my wounds (putting pressure on the cuts to stop the bleeding) I was also thinking about the ontological 'situation' that I was experiencing and how I was trying to make sense of my enfleshed body that was actually leaking in front of me. I was also thinking about how I should be reacting and presenting myself within this situation.

The session started pretty well. It was my regular Friday session with (my trainer) and during the previous week he had been competing in a large competition and, after having experienced the events, had returned with a number of ideas about how to change both his training and mine. He had been quite surprised about the volume of training that was needed, especially after having spoken to other competitors about the amount of training that they were doing. When he had asked them about how much training they do most were doing several sessions a day, while coach JP had been doing five sessions per week. Subsequently he felt that we needed to be doing more and so on his return he had revised my training schedule so that I could build more sessions during the week. I don't really mind doing more and I like having a structure to follow. The sessions that I had completed by myself on Monday and Wednesday this week had been tougher, but I could see the benefit of gradually pushing the intensity. The one on Wednesday was especially tough as I had to do a final WoD which was a timed session consisting of 100×40 kg back squats, 50 push-ups and 25 pullups. I had initially thought the hundred back squats would be really challenging but when I did do them I found that by pacing myself and breaking them up strategically I could get through them without difficulty. The next day, however, my legs were really sore. They haven't been like this for a long time and while it felt satisfying that I had really done something and the evidence of my effort was apparent in the soreness, I was fairly tired when it came to the session on Friday. I suppose the thing I have to realise as well is that when coach JP was talking to these other competitors it is difficult to know what else they are during the day. Do they have full-time jobs? If they do, how are they really able to do five sessions a day?

So, although I was feeling tired as well as sore in my legs I was still thinking that it would be good to do the session and that I would feel better afterwards. Also, I had in the back of my mind that I would have the weekend free anyway to recover.

The session started really well and we talked about the new schedule and then went into a warm-up routine which was followed by a series of Olympic lifting practices.

(I shouldn't really mention this on the blog, as I know that coach JP reads it, but I actually really enjoy the Olympic lifting. I don't think I'm very good, but I know I'm getting better and that is satisfying. I say this because there are some mind games going on and I'm going to write about this in the next blog post. Because I know that if I say I like something or I mention that I find something relatively easy, I'm pretty sure that he will increase the weight or add to the intensity. So I'm learning to be pretty cagey about what I do reveal!)

Anyhow, after the initial warm-ups and practice we moved on to the WOD. This was going to be a timed activity which included rounds of cleans, deadlifts and box jumps. We had a practice of each of the exercises and this included some box jumps. I was quite pleased that I could do the 30-inch box, especially after struggling over the last couple of years with a meniscus injury. However, for this WoD, coach

JP thought the 24-inch would be better as the jumps would get harder later on in the session.

The WOD started well. I completed the cleans and then the deadlifts. At this stage, I was probably a little too eager to complete the round and instead of moving to the box step and positioning myself for the jump, I cut that corner and went straight into the first jump. I think because I was too far away, my feet only touched the side of the box step and in doing so slipped back off the edge leaving me to do a belly flop onto the box. During the fall I managed to scrape every part of my body on the wooden edges as I wrapped myself round the box step.

At first I thought I would carry on until I noticed my legs bleeding. My reaction as well as coach JP's was to just have a quick break, mop up the blood and then continue. However, while he went off to get some plasters, I noticed more grazes on my thighs and arms. I sat down and attempted to mop up the blood on my legs with the T-shirt I had discarded earlier in the session. By that time I started to feel a little shaky and when coach JP returned with the first aid kit we realised that it wouldn't be a good idea to carry on. Apart from the physical pain (signalling to me that my body had been hurt), I felt annoyed that I had fallen, as well as slightly cheated that I couldn't continue the session. Falling over was just SO inconvenient!

It was interesting, however, the thoughts that went through my head while I was sitting there with bleeding legs. When coach JP came back with the first aid kit, he also had some paper towels to wipe the blood away. It made me think about social attitudes to blood. In this case it was my blood and for coach JP it was someone else's blood. Obviously, these things happen all the time, but in this instance the body is transformed into something 'other' especially in relation to how it was understood only a few minutes previously. I'm thinking here about the transition from an able, performing body to an 'injured' one that is not able anymore. While, in this particular case, my injury is probably only considered by everyone involved in terms of being a temporary event, the presence of blood was a stark reminder of a corporeal body that is fragile and could be damaged. This fragile body is in total contrast to the perception of a strong, capable and almost 'immortal' body that is performed in the everyday routines of CrossFit and most sports for that matter.

My bleeding legs also made me think about the social context of blood and the places in which it is acceptable. I've seen the rhetoric used to promote CrossFit as an activity where blood and sweat are the bywords for anyone who is 'serious' about the sport. At this stage, I'm not really sure how I relate to this. Maybe I have passed some form of rite of passage, although it wasn't intentional and if that is the case, once is enough for me, thank-you.

Third week—pain in perspective

I don't really want this to be a blog about pain although, at this stage, it does seem like it is rapidly moving in that direction. It will be interesting to see how much it does dominate over the next few months and maybe my current preoccupation with it will diminish as it becomes something of an everyday occurrence and my body becomes more accustomed to it. However, at the moment I am still really aware of the different forms of pain and exhaustion that I'm experiencing and having to negotiate. I am also aware of how I can capture, record and try to understand it, because the intense feelings that I experience during the activities are really complex and I am aware that the time that lapses between the actual experience and how I set about reflecting upon and recording it may impact upon how accurately I can remember them or reflect upon it in sufficient detail. Nevertheless, sitting here now and shutting my eyes in an attempt to remember those experiences from the last session on Saturday, the memories are still vivid, so I want to try to document these. I am also thinking about maybe using a video camera to record some of my future sessions so that afterwards I can look back at what I was doing and try to provide a narrative as I watch.

For now, what I'm trying to do here is take into consideration how it is always easy to sit back after the event and develop a rational explanation for what happened during it. In this case, I am trying to make sense of the way that I experience things like pain, discomfort and exhaustion for what really is only a brief period of time—but, in these moments, seem like the only time that there is in the world. I know that doesn't make complete sense—but it is something I have become aware of during the intense period that occurs when the body is pushed physically and emotionally in the latter stages of a WoD. Here there is no time or space during the actual experience to attempt to understand it, while afterwards is a time to try to put these feelings into some sort of perspective. In this post I am concentrating upon the WoD that I undertook at the end of last Saturday's session with coach JP. During that session, there were a range of pre-planned activities coach JP had prepared. This was my third session with him since starting the training and I have been following his planned sessions during the week. As usual, before we started the WoD there were some warm-up activities and coaching of techniques related to different forms of lifting. The final activity was the WoD, which comprised a timed activity of the following exercises:

(Four rounds of)

Bear crawl (length of 20-metre hall and back)

21 thrusters (20-kg bar)

15 kb swings (20 kg)

9 crunches (on rings)

Once again the session appeared to be designed to play tricks on the body. 20-kg is not particularly heavy, but when one gets used to doing a set of 10 or 12 repetitions, 21 suddenly adds another dimension to this. Combined with the rounds being continuous (with no rest between sets, like in conventional weight training) the routine becomes more challenging. Also, I didn't really take into account the bear crawl to start with. I had initially thought of it something like a jog up the hall and back. Although after the first round, it felt considerably more exhausting than the stroll that I had first envisaged.

Being timed also added to the tension and I was aware of the clock ticking down right from the start. I can remember thinking that I mustn't look at it so that I could fully concentrate and not preoccupy myself with how much time I had left and whether I could keep going. In theory, I should really carry on until I heard the final beep and I should let coach JP shout out how long I had, if he felt I needed to know. However, the sensible approach was easier said than done. I felt like Orpheus, in that once I had been told (albeit by myself) not to look at the clock I felt compelled to do so. The clock was my Eurydice and I had to look back. From then on the gates of Hades opened further and I was plunged into more turmoil—both physical and mental.

I know this sounds a bit dramatic, but my intensive sensations of exhaustion are interesting to unpack further (especially from the comfort of my chair after I have had time to recover). As I mentioned in my last post the word 'pain' does not sufficiently account for the embodied feeling that I experience. It is an intensive exhaustion that closes out everything else around me. In this case, all I could see was the bar in front of me and that all my focus was upon lifting it above my head for a few more times. It was an existential moment, in that nothing else mattered. I wasn't, however, 'in the zone' because I was aware of coach JP shouting out encouragement. Time had frozen in some way for me in terms of my existential being at that moment, although, contradictorily, I was aware of the clock ticking and the movement of time, by my awareness that I only had a little time left.

In this moment, my shoulders and arms were 'in pain', but this was a pain related to fatigue and a feeling that I had no more strength or energy left to be able to push the bar above my head. These feelings were being encouraged by voices in my head saying that I couldn't do any more and I should stop. However, I wanted to do more and I could hear coach JP saying I could do more ('only two more'—'come on, push through'). This makes me think that in that moment, I was not in a complete existential vacuum because I could sense coach JP's presence. Maybe because of that, I had to negotiate not only physical fatigue but also my awareness of the possibility of failure—and what that would mean in terms of what I have staked in this embodied project (and my own feelings of self-worth).

It was strange that it seemed like only a few minutes later I was sitting chatting to coach JP about the workout. We talked about those intense feelings of exhaustion and how a lot of it was about controlling those negative voices. I thought then that if I could remember during those really intense moments of exhaustion I would be feel fine immediately after it might help overcome the voices saying 'I can't do any more'. Whether I can get to the stage of actually remembering this during those moments is another matter—watch this space.

Fun and games

During the first month or so I have been more preoccupied with learning about what CrossFit is about and whether my body can actually deliver what the sport and I am demanding from it. Because of this, maybe unsurprisingly, the focus of my posts (or thoughts) has been on things like physical pain and exhaustion as well as my feelings related to whether I am or can be good enough to continue.

It might be the case that as I have now had time to get into the training process more I have been able to recognise other factors that make up the whole package of CrossFit (and any other sport for that matter) and, in particular, I have become more aware of the pleasurable aspects of the activities. In the last couple sessions with coach JP we have been incorporating a range of activities and, on reflection, these have made me think more about what it was that made these activities enjoyable and why some have been more enjoyable than others. As I have detailed in previous posts, certain aspects of the activities can produce differing responses. Some might be more influenced by my physical ability to do them, my perceptions of the activity beforehand, how I am feeling on that day and so on. However, I was aware during my last session with coach JP that it was 'fun' rather than in previous WoDs where the focus was very much upon completing the task—and where enjoyment would be experienced after the event. The session was not as physically intense as some of the others and it might be that in the more intensive activities exhaustion temporarily distracts from immediate feelings of enjoyment. However, it did dawn on me that

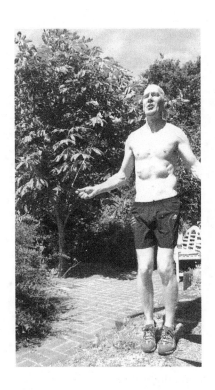

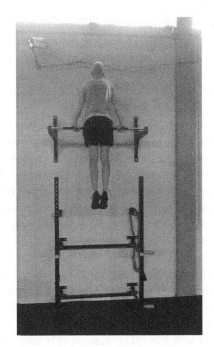

FIGURE 4.2 Examples of physical play *(continued)*

(continued)

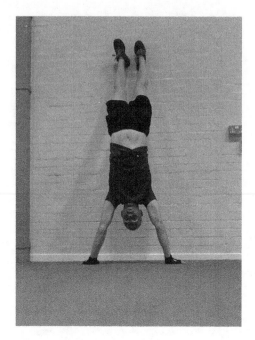

FIGURE 4.2 Examples of physical play

much of my enjoyment was a result of the activities being almost like play sessions. Now that I was starting to get the 'hang of' CrossFit, the play aspect was becoming more apparent. It seems like there are lots of activities that are pretty much like adult (or not so adult) versions of childhood play. Things like climbing on bars, skipping, running, jumping, doing handstands and so on.

The session itself started with a series of warm-ups, then a section of instruction based upon overhead squatting techniques. I am also enjoying the learning aspects of the sessions. It is satisfying to have time to concentrate on specific aspects and workout how to develop technique. Overhead squatting is something that I need to work on. It is taking a while for my body (specifically my shoulders) to recalibrate after years of playing tennis and being hunched over a computer. So, while my general flexibility is pretty good my Achilles heel at the moment is the lack of mobility in my shoulders, which is in turn affecting my range of movement in the overhead squat. Recognising this as a challenge and, subsequently, developing a strategy to work on it is satisfying—although equally frustrating during the early stages of attempting the movements.

The main WoD was the 'play' session this time. It consisted of 4 rounds of timed sprints with each round comprising four 20-metre sprints—with a burpee after each 20 metres. 2 minutes was allocated for each round so that there would be an element of recovery after a round. The intention was for each round of sprints to be completed in the same time. It worked out that I was doing each one in about 20 seconds.

Although the times were important as well as learning about the importance of pacing and recovery, what I really enjoyed most was just 'running' and jumping on to the mat at the end of each 20 metres. It seemed like ages since I had done anything like this. It was fun and although it did have a purpose in the overall scheme of my training, I did like that it provided legitimate opportunities for fun and games and, ultimately, the chance to act like a 'kid' again.

5

EMBODIED PLEASURE AND PAIN IN FITNESS-RELATED PRACTICES

> It is a messy process, involving a vast number of different, even contradictory language games, cognitive processes, affective practices, and motivations. This should not surprise us. After all, pain is a type of event that involves not only sensation, but also cognition, affect, and motivational aspects. Meanings, history, learning, and expectations all influence ways of being-in-pain.
>
> *(Bourke 2014, p. 301)*

In the introduction I talked about some of my early memories of childhood and teenage years and how all those experiences contributed to an embodied self that did not have cause to contemplate health as anything other than unproblematic. (Good) health and being able to move my body in the way that I wanted it to was never in question. I cannot really remember any periods during my childhood when I was ill and find it hard to pinpoint a time when I can remember being incapacitated, apart from on one occasion when I broke my arm and another when I had to have my appendix removed. These were only temporary aberrations and were merely considered inconvenient in that they forced me to be inactive for a very brief period of time. All the while I knew that I would be getting better soon. Experience of, and not really having any direct contact with, unhealthy bodies created an obliviousness or complacency (or lack of consciousness) about unhealthiness. Indeed, health was not even a factor to be contemplated because I had no reason to question it.

The reason for highlighting my lack of awareness suggests to me that for many the notion of ill-health is not a problem unless there is some direct confrontation with it. However, there are other factors involved here. Although I did not experience significant physical exposure to ill-health in my youth, it could also be suggested that as a 'healthy and active young man' it created little need for me to have to consider and negotiate health, or the notion of ill-health. Indeed, the social perception of a young man in contemporary western society is generally co-terminous with what healthy should look like. My awareness of youth and gender discourses became apparent only through my later studies in sociology. It was then that I could understand the different social requirements relating to outward performances of a gendered and youthful body. More specifically, the significance of broader social discourses on women's bodies, and how my naturalised formulation of a healthy body and absence of discussion about potential ill-health or the limitations of a physical body, was in contrast to those experienced by women, particularly during and after puberty in terms of the effect that awareness of a physical, sexual, reproductive body had on later physical identity (de Beauvoir 1972, Firestone 1979).

Although my enhanced awareness of how others may experience their bodies was developed through academic study and could be considered a form of enlightenment, those years of complacency about my healthy body make it difficult to completely disassociate myself from the formation of a sense of indestructability or immunity—in that I still harbour delusions that I have and always will have a healthy body.

I mention this because it is difficult to completely absolve myself from those formative years of body fascism (albeit unintentional body fascism). The unconscious contemplation of my body in a specific way has forged a sense of self that is physically able and in possession of a body that can move about in relatively unrestricted ways. Unbeknown at the time, and as feminist academics have argued, my ability to be expressive with my body has been significantly enhanced by social constructions of gender that promote the active, moving male body in contrast to the inactive, passive female body (Young 1980, Hargreaves 1994, Segal 1997). As Connell (1995) argues, in her descriptions of masculinities, I have at times been unwittingly complicit in the reinforcement of gender binaries, precisely because I had little, if any, reason to question the status quo.

I can say that I was lucky. However, I am not proposing that I should not have been lucky, but rather that those opportunities made available to me should have been available to all. As a child I did not have any sense of my complicity in reinforcing gender binaries. Why would I? I was not exposed to any forms of thought that challenged the existing social structure. Nevertheless, I hope that if I had been offered alternative ways of thinking I would have been amenable to them.

My reason for mentioning these points relating to gender here is that I am incorporating a similar approach to thinking about the moving body. As I have described in Chapter 3, the embodied approach that informs the discussion throughout the book draws on the notion of body-reflexive practices that are central to our formulation of our selves. In the same way that acknowledging the influence of social constructionist theory helps us contest the inequalities found in established (heteronormative) accounts of gender, so too do we need to recognise the ways in which the social body shapes our contemplation of the moving body.

Although I am mindful of the significant contribution that post-structural theory has made to our understanding of the discourses that operate to control and organise our bodies, I am also aware of the shortfall that such discursively centred theorising creates. This shortfall is possibly generated through a methodological stance that by necessity concentrates on the discursive structures of language. In doing so, although bodies may be the subject of scrutiny, they are, nevertheless, abstract bodies in text. For instance, Foucault made a point of attempting to distance himself from the theory and separate his personal life (as such his own body) from the texts he was studying. This lack of embodied reflexivity is called into question when one considers that in his personal life he had to negotiate homosexuality (which was stigmatised and criminalised for a significant period of his life), actively embraced a sexually charged gay scene in San Francisco and battled AIDS-related ill-health in his final years (Miller 1994). All of this not only must have affected his embodied identity, but also equally contributed to the questions that he felt needed exploring. Although the decision to keep his private life separate from his public academic role may have been fuelled by attempts to adopt scientific rigour, expected within academia, it is still difficult to reconcile how his personal embodied experiences could not enter into his thought processes. Thus, Foucault's attempts to address a 'will to truth' (adapted from Nietzsche's [1969] initial concept), in which the quest for truth was ultimately influenced by different historical formulations of philosophy, religion, morals and science, ultimately need some form of reflexive consideration of the writer within this analysis. Consequently, although the initial approach to focus on the structures that have a bearing on the individual creates the need to pay attention to the ways in which knowledge is constructed through language, it does not mean we should ignore the way in which the individual acts on and experiences knowledge through the body. Butler (1997) does take an extra step towards acknowledging the body by drawing on personal experience of alternative sexuality.

As a gay woman, she reflects upon personal experience in order to question the complex ways in which gay people respond to their sexuality. She describes how she 'sought to understand some of the terror and anxiety that some people suffer in "becoming gay"' (Butler 1997, p. xi). Although the condition of being gay is understood in terms of the social regimes of signification that describe it, the notion of 'terror' suggests a much greater embodied experience, but does not fully account for the participation in the physical experience that caused the terror and anxiety suffered by the individual. Terror and anxiety also relate to a bodily terror and I am reminded of the way that Sartre (1956) described how the impact of becoming aware of one's existence (and meaninglessness) affects thoughts, ideas and feelings, as well as the physical body through an embodied feeling of nausea. Terror (or nausea) is at the same time a psychological and physiological manifestation that acts on the body.

Consequently, bearing in mind the terror that Butler describes in relation to an individual's recognition of a socially perceived 'deviant' sexuality, how does this equate with a writer (Foucault) who actively embraced socially taboo sexual practices? How could these not influence the orientation, disposition and emotional reaction to the knowledge that he was exploring? Although I am not disputing the significance of his work, I find it difficult to see how he could conduct a personal life that would have exposed him to a range of embodied sensations without it having an impact on how he reflected upon and negotiated his intellectual writing. I am not suggesting that Foucault did not consider these, but it was his ultimate methodological decision to exclude the embodied aspects of his own life and how they contribute to his thought processes that leaves unanswered questions. These have been more successfully accommodated in feminist theories (such as Butler 1993, Phipps 2014), which have adopted post-structural perspectives, as well as more recent phenomenological feminist thinking (Allen-Collinson & Owton 2015). Here there is greater emphasis on the female body as one that has been subjected to disadvantage because of essentialist descriptions of a biological body that is different to a male's. Recognition of the biological body provides a mechanism to challenge the supposed scientific 'truths' about the superiority of the male. Feminist writers can clearly be seen to have employed a form of embodiedness in the way that they incorporated personal experience of the body, particularly a sexual, reproductive body, that was subjugated because of its biological difference to the male counterpart.

Nevertheless, mindful as I am about the social influence of discourses of knowledge, I cannot overlook the significance of the physical experience and how it may interconnect with or remain separate from the social description (or discourse). For example, an orgasm is an orgasm if viewed in terms of a physical experience. However, if we factor in the social and cultural understanding of it, along with when, where and how it occurs (and whether alone or with another), this creates a multitude of possible experiences that may affect the physical sensation as well as the social reaction. Consequently, it is with a body-reflexive lens that I contemplate the notion of pleasure and pain as it has emerged, not only in Chapter 4, but in earlier writing (Wellard 2013), as a significant factor in the way that a sporting or physical activity is experienced. Although I was aware that pain and pleasure would be evident throughout the period of intensive training, the extent to which it did remain such a dominant theme in my reflections, and manifested in ways that I was not always expecting, was still surprising. To an extent, I could not escape from it and I needed to document those experiences so that I could attempt to understand it in more depth.

At the same time, other experiences, such as undergoing surgery on my eye, provided an opportunity to reflect further about the context of pain and the situations in which one might be justified in incorporating pleasure with pain and others where there would be little resonance. This may explain my critique of Foucault in that there is a disparity between the sophisticated theory that he offers and the disembodied detachment that is apparent in the light of many accounts about his personal life and apparent experimentation with extreme sexual practices (Miller 1994). Whether the stories about his delving into sadomasochism are exaggerated, it still suggests that there were opportunities for him to explore an embodied existence in more depth. Although I can see the potential for participation in sadomasochistic practices as an area that may offer opportunities to explore ideas beyond the limits of conventional embodied experiences, I am a little too squeamish to follow that route. Nevertheless, this may explain my reference to the performance artist, ORLAN, in Chapter 4, and the possibilities for using the body as a project for developing thinking. Although her methodological approach in using her own body as the subject of her art may be at the opposite end of the spectrum in relation to Foucault, it does provide an interesting comparison. My reference to her may have initially been somewhat flippant, but there are elements that resonate with my attempts to incorporate my own body into the study, in ways that I had not contemplated before, in order to be able to address and contemplate some of the methodological gaps remaining in post-structural theorising.

What follows, then, is a more detailed focus on the theme of pain and enjoyment that I highlighted in Chapter 4—in this case, a consideration of the way in which pain is experienced at both the social and physical levels. At the same time, the reflections that I have included also draw attention to the notion of shared pain and pleasure as well as personal pain and the pain of others. For example, after I had completed the intensive training period, I continued to train and take part in competitions (see Chapter 6 for an account of my embracing a CrossFit identity). On one occasion, I took part in a competition with a colleague which involved completing a series of activities that were recorded and timed. In each activity one completed the task while the other recorded and offered encouragement. I went first and experienced the intense exhaustive pain that taking part entailed. In the same way that I described the training activities in Chapter 4, I found ways to manage the feelings of pain and exhaustion as I strived to finish in the quickest time possible. Throughout I was aware of my colleague shouting encouragement, but at the time could focus only on each movement required. When I had finished, I watched my colleague doing the same event. However, even though I knew exactly what he was going through, I found his presentations of agony (grunts/grimaces) amusing. Even with the knowledge that I had just been through the same ordeal, I could not associate the same levels of empathy, as if his pain was not as 'real' as what I had just been through.

I have included this example, because it implies that there is even greater complexity in the way that we can describe and understand the experience of pain. However, before I attempt to consider this further, it is important to consider the ways in which knowledge about pain has been generated.

As Anthony Synnott (1993) describes, the body has been contemplated in a range of ways throughout history. Similarly, Joanna Bourke (2014) reveals the contrasting ways that pain has been understood during different historical eras. What this tells us is that pain is not only a subjective physical sensation in a purely individual way but also that it is dynamic in that it can be interpreted differently at a social level at different socio-historical times. As such, external influences through which the individual can learn to experience pain (or indeed pleasure) in a totally different way need to be recognised. Thus, my reflections upon the experiences of pain and intensive exhaustion can be compared with other subjective accounts, such as Atkinson's (2010) descriptions of his pleasurable suffering while engaging in fell running, in order to understand the significance of multiple factors that have created these experiences over a period of time.

Bourke provides an extensive account of the history of social understanding of pain. Her focus is on the broader general interpretation of pain in terms of suffering and its relationship to the human condition.

Although the way in which I want to explore pain and pleasure is within the context of sport and physical activity, Bourke's work is important here because it provides further evidence of the competing and arbitrary ways in which pain can be understood, and how we need to recognise the relevance and input of socio-cultural and historical constructions of how pain might be experienced.

Particularly relevant to my discussion in this book is Bourke's description of how diagnosing pain has been accommodated within medical discourse, and how this has influenced the ways in which we might seek to describe a painful experience as well as the way that these formulations generate templates for how we might provide descriptions of levels of pain. Not only is this relevant in terms of demonstrating the varying and subjective nature of describing pain, but it also draws attention to the mechanisms that have heavily influenced scientific approaches to studying and classifying pain, which have, in turn, been adopted by a range of complementary and competing groups.

Bourke describes how, within medical sites, the formulation of the McGill Pain Questionnaire[1] provided a way of using language (in terms of descriptions of pain) to assist medical practitioners with their diagnoses of illness and disease. However, as Bourke notes, there remains a cultural specificity with many pain descriptors. She provides an example of experts of pain language from three different cultures (English, Finnish and Japanese) who argued that culture and language not only affect thought and cognition, but also may affect the actual experience of pain (Bourke 2014, p. 151).

For Bourke (2014, p. 151), 'being in pain might FEEL different in different cultures', whereas the same may be claimed about the experiences of individuals in similar cultures but at different historical periods. According to her:

> If culture (including language) and physiology are in constant dynamic interaction, we would expect to see differences not only between eighteenth-century sufferers and their twenty-first-century counterparts, but also between distinctive natural or geographic groups.
>
> *(Bourke 2014, p. 151)*

Similar to Synnott (1993) in his analysis of the social body, Bourke can chart the way that pain has been understood historically in multiple ways and, in so doing, highlights the significance of social and cultural interpretation, rather than just of purely scientifically based, physiological explanations. The socio-cultural context is clearly integral to how we might formulate an understanding of the body in pain (or pleasure). Consequently, bearing this in mind, a move into the more specific realm of sport and physical activity presents even further layers of interpretation.

It could be suggested that, within the context of sport and physical activity, pain has been considered in more pragmatic ways, where it is to be managed for greater performance rather than as a reflection of the human condition or wider social suffering. Sport, particularly performance sport, operates with a much more utilitarian approach in that it regards the body in terms of a mechanical tool that needs to be fine-tuned. However, there is a learning process that is also incorporated—one in which understanding about the body needs to be seen in terms of developing a 'feel' for the body. However, rather than offering exciting possibilities for generating a sense of existential embodiedness, this sense of feeling is more akin to that of a racing driver getting a feel for the car and how the engine works. There is a distinct level of detachment in this process and it echoes broader knowledge about the body based on the Cartesian mind/body dualism that is so entrenched in contemporary thinking. This separated mind/body understanding maintains a detached approach to the body where it contemplated, similar to a car, the individual (mind) as the driver.

In sport the management of pain presents athletes (drivers) with a requirement that they must be alert to how their body responds when it needs to perform. Consequently, athletes need to learn how their body reacts to pain to be able to perform at intense levels, and then recognise when it is appropriate to push their body further (or through pain). Knowledge developed about different 'types' of pain creates the notion of positive pain (or Zátopekian pain), and introduces to the athlete an expectation that there are and will be different levels of pain and, in simple terms, the need to distinguish between good pain and bad pain. Positive (good) pain is often considered in terms of how to describe the fatigue that an elite sporting participant goes through in the process of trying to enhance performance. Therefore, any properly structured athletic training should be developed to maximise this component of pain, in other words the notion of a 'no pain, no gain' culture (Stamford 1987). The logic here is that, by exposing sporting participants to pain, while they are injury free, the process of training is believed to raise their pain threshold (Carmichael 1988). Pain is considered to be constructive if incorporated in periods of intense training that are followed by no negative side effects from training and/or involvement in competition or performance.

In this interpretation, pain is understood in terms of fatigue and muscle soreness, which are quite different from overtraining or staleness, although they may exist during such states. These are considered 'everyday' aspects of training but are, nevertheless, an essential aspect of participation.

Zátopekian pain is therefore considered to be positive, in that fatigue and muscle soreness will be inevitable, but also an expected outcome or indication of hard work and effort during training. In this way, Zátopekian pain or positive pain is considered as to be an aspect of training that will help to increase the body's immunity to pain and the pain threshold. Pickard (2007), in her study of young ballet dancers, demonstrated how learning about good and bad pain was a central aspect of dancers' training, to the extent that they developed an enhanced awareness of 'types' of pain. For example, in her interviews with the dancers, one 14-year-old dancer described her understanding of muscle soreness:

> Sometimes my body gets so tired and it aches and I think 'I'll never do anymore' but I do and I feel good. You have to find the determination to do the best you can, you want to prove yourself all the time, to push all the time, sometimes a little 'cos you're scared about how much it is going to hurt but you realise there's more there and it's ok. You might be stiff but you know eventually it'll wear off. You push through it and gain that much more.
> *(Female ballet dancer, aged 14, quoted in Pickard 2007, p. 45)*

For any sports or dance performers, it is the expectation that they will (have to) develop the ability to distinguish between types of pain so that they can identify potential injury or push their training harder. It is interesting that this could be considered as a form of embodied awareness that is consciously considered, although it is probably not articulated by coaches in this way. Either way, it is also significant that the coach plays a role in the process. Pickard also acknowledged the part that the trainer has in encouraging such embodied awareness as well as being equally important in observing and guarding their students from pushing too far.

> They have to learn what pain they can work through and what hurts. I think stretching is a nice pain but they don't all seem to. When they say 'ow!' we have to work out if it is that the muscles really aren't going to do it and are in danger of snapping or whether it is just that they have to get used to that feeling of lengthening. Most children would have been through a certain

amount of pain to get here anyway so therefore they should know themselves if it's a nice hurt or if it's an agony. I think most of the pain is good and as dancers you expect pain to be good and doing good. It is difficult with children though as their bones are growing and not their muscles.

(Ballet teacher, quoted in Pickard 2007, p. 46)

The embodied aspects of engaging in sport automatically create an orientation to the body that is not just about one's own body, but also accommodates the environment and other bodies, whether or not directly involved. It is an ontological situation that incorporates, drawing on Sartre (1956), an embodied sense of being for oneself and being for others.

Consequently, there are, of necessity, relationships with the self and others that need to be assessed, interpreted, negotiated and acted on. The arguments about relationships of power that Foucault (1978, 1979) puts forward are significant here, especially in terms of the complexity of the way in which they manifest themselves, as well as in the way that relationships are recognised as being both an internal relationship with the individual body and one with external bodies. However, as much as these resonate with the themes being explored in this book, my methodological approach has been informed bearing in mind Connell's (1995) body-reflexive practices, which are formed through a range of embodied experiences that link to bodily interaction and bodily experience via socially constructed bodily understandings, which in turn lead to new bodily interactions. As a result of this, Connell suggests that social theory needs to provide more recognition for the corporeality of the body. It is 'through body-reflexive practices, bodies are addressed by social process and drawn into history, without ceasing to be bodies. . . . they do not turn into symbols, signs or positions in discourse' (Connell 1995, p. 64).

Connell's concept of body-reflexive practices is, therefore, helpful in that it highlights how social and cultural factors interact with individual experiences of the body. This reveals not only the social forms and practices that underpin the individual's ability to take part in sport, dance and physical activity, but also the unique experiences or physical thrill of embodied expression. As discussed in Chapter 3, I adapted the concept to assist my understanding of the embodied experiences of pleasure within the context of sport and physical activities. I described this as a circuit of body-reflexive pleasures and, within this context, if we apply the concept to an individual's experience of a sport, we can see that consideration needs to be made of the social, physiological and psychological processes that occur at any level and with varied influences. An important aspect of this theorisation was the acknowledgement of temporal and spatial factors within the circuit because these provide a response to claims that pleasure is a 'one-off', insignificant, moment of self-gratification precisely because it is part of a complex extended process in which a pleasurable experience also has a before and an after. For example, an activity may be experienced several times before it is considered as pleasurable, or may be experienced in a space that shifts the dynamics of the circuit, such as the social and physical 'space' where the experience occurs (for instance, a gym, a CrossFit 'box' or a public park). In this way, the additional acknowledgement of time and space highlights how pleasure can be seen to be connected with geographical aspects of both personal experiences and social encounters. Consequently, the circuit describes pleasure in terms of a continually 'moving' process which includes elements of anticipation, experience and reflection.

Incorporating temporal dimensions also helps with accounting for the process of age. Thus, rather than as only a social factor of a specific physiological stage, the notion of a constantly changing body that is ageing makes us consider a further cog in the circuit. For example, if we take the experience of an elderly amateur sportsperson and an elite athlete participating in a marathon run, how they experience the activity will be determined by a circuit of body-reflexive practices that will produce different physical reactions and feelings precisely because of the various competing social, psychological and physical factors at play. In this way, the experience of the activity (and their levels of intensity or engagement) will be influenced by a range of contrasting factors, such as the initial orientation to the activity (professional, career, fun runner, novice, experienced), self-identity, physiological conditioning, expectations, goals and so on, This suggests that social factors interact with individual experiences of the body and signal the need to recognise not only the social forms and practices that underpin the individual's ability to take part in sport or physical activity, but also the unique experiences or physical thrill of bodily based expression. Consequently, although social codes may dictate to the individual the appropriateness of taking part in an organized sport event, it does not necessarily take into account how the individual enjoys the experience.

In order to explore body-reflexive pleasures further and, indeed, draw attention to the socio-cultural aspects that contribute to how a physical activity such as CrossFit training is experienced, I have included two themes from Chapter 4 that were significant in the overall experience. These relate to the notion of intensive exhaustion and fun and games.

Intensive exhaustion

The example of taking part in an intense physical activity reveals not only the highly personal experiences that combine physiological and psychological reactions but also, in this case, the difficulties in attempting to understand and then make generalisations about what the experience may look and feel like. Consequently, when I attempted to describe the experiences of undergoing the training sessions and workouts, I had to bear in mind the interpretations of pain that have already been offered. The notion of pain in terms of suffering in the way that Bourke describes, or the medicalised version of pain that relates to an injury, does not provide sufficient recognition of the context in which this 'pain' occurred. The pain that I experience is neither related to suffering caused through human inequality and injustice nor a medical condition that causes incapacity. I choose to do the activity and choose to continue with the activity even though my body is hurting. In this case there is a possibility that I have learnt to distinguish between good and bad pain, as mentioned above. It might also suggest that I have managed to move into some form of transcendental space where it is possible to negotiate the intensive exhaustion that I describe.

> [T]he word 'pain' does not sufficiently account for the embodied feeling that I experience. It is an intensive exhaustion that closes out everything else around me. In this case, all I could see was the bar in front of me and that all my focus was upon lifting it above my head for a few more times. It was an existential moment, in that nothing else mattered. I wasn't, however, 'in the zone' because I was aware of coach JP shouting out encouragement. Time had frozen in some way for me in terms of my existential being at that moment, although, contradictorily, I was aware of the clock ticking and the movement of time, by my awareness that I only had a little time left.

In this case, I mentioned the notion of getting into a zone, which implies some form of embodied transcendence. Indeed, Pronger (2002, p. 8) also mentioned in his discussion of technologies of fitness that 'there is little theorizing on the horizons of transcendence in modern body culture'. Most discussion about being in the zone has been found within sports performance, especially within psychology, as a means of understanding how an individual responds to an altered mental state, (Csikszentmihalyi 1990). However, there remain absences in terms of accounting for what is 'going on' around the individual and how these contributing factors create an environment where entering the zone might be possible, as reflected in the account above of what I was and was not aware of around me.

Woodward (2015) contributes to the discussion by incorporating a socio-cultural perspective. She describes the 'enfleshed' aspects of being in the zone, which provides a useful way to unravel some of these complexities because it includes a sense of 'movement' in and out of consciousness and, importantly, how it is more than an individual 'state of mind'. Consequently, where the concept of being in the zone has been developed predominantly through psychological theorisation, in particular within the context of performance-based activities such as elite sport and professional music, the focus for such research has tended to concentrate on how an individual might be able to harness such a state of mind to improve performance. However, the accounts of movement experiences in the context of sport, as described in the extract above, reveal a form of 'transcendence' that is not fully explained through traditional versions of being in the zone. This example of an embodied sporting experience in CrossFit is often replicated in other sporting activities, for instance, fell running (Atkinson 2015) and surfing (Evers 2015) and might initially be explained in terms of occasions where getting into a zone occurred. However, they also provide examples of embodied 'movement' experienced as both physical and social. In doing so, they reveal forms of transcendence that need to be understood within the context of the environment and the socio-political influences that created such spaces as CrossFit, fell-running and surfing.

A criticism often levelled at purely psychological analyses of being in the zone is that explanations offered are based on assumptions of a mind and body binary. By attempting to move beyond mind–body dualisms, embodied approaches allow the research process to accommodate movement between states of being that are not only about perception but also just as much about the embodied experience. Thus, my reflections on the training sessions reveal the embodied experiences of taking part in an activity and offer 'fleshed-out' detail of what is or can be experienced. In many cases, these accounts describe how one can become 'seduced' by an activity or get 'caught up in the moment'. This notion of getting caught up suggests some form of movement of conscious being and resonates with the original premise that an individual moves into the 'zone'. However, as Woodward (2015) points out, thinking about transcendence in this case is not only about a psychological state but an experience that physically takes over the body. One does not enter into a virtual reality (like some form of computer game) but simultaneously one encounters the experience as a social and physical event. For instance:

I could hear coach JP saying I could do more ('only two more'—'come on, push through'). This makes me think that in that moment, I was not in a complete existential vacuum because I could sense coach JP's presence. Maybe because of that, I had to negotiate not only physical fatigue but also my awareness of the possibility of failure—and what that would mean in terms of what I have staked in this embodied project (and my own feelings of self-worth).

Importantly, experiences such as the one described here suggest that it is not only the individual who is affected in the zone but also others (in this case the coach) who are in the immediate environment because the individual does not become invisible to the rest of the world. (Indeed, it could be argued that the immediate environment could also include a virtual reality created through live social media.) In this way, unlike the general discussion on 'flow', which tends to be based on the positive effects of being in the zone (because of the focus on elite performance), there is a tendency to overlook what is happening 'outside' the zone, and the possible beneficial or harmful effects that the individual 'in' the zone may have on other people (for example, an over-zealous boxer or an over-competitive sports person).

Just like attempting to create a 'one size fits all' description of pain, the notion of being in the zone is, indeed, more complicated when taking into account the broader dimensions of socio-cultural factors, as well as embodied experiences of intense forms of physical activity in sport. Whether the reflections that I provide in this book can fit neatly into established definitions of what being in the zone should look like is not entirely clear. The research aims for this book were not about exploring the experience of being in a zone. However, themes that emerged relating to transcendence, movement into 'other' forms of consciousness and embodied experiences of pleasure and pain suggested similar characteristics of entering into a 'zone'. Consequently, I have attempted to use these examples as a means of 'troubling' (Butler 1990) conventional explanations of bitz by highlighting the less than straightforward movement into a zone. In particular, these examples provide support for Woodward's (2015) argument that bitz needs to be understood in terms of more complex movements in and out of 'consciousness'

Focus on the embodied experiences of pleasure and pain reveals the importance of recognising the context of where bitz occurs and the activity that is producing it. In the social context of CrossFit (as well as other forms of sporting and dance activities), a simplistic pain/pleasure dichotomy is inadequate because bodily limits are explored out of an apparent desire by the participant to do so, in order to move beyond the normal or previous self. In the original concept of 'flow' (Csikszentmihalyi 1990), pleasure and fun were described as a consequence in relation to motivation. Pleasure was generally dismissed because it was considered merely as a conscious state when a need is satisfied, whereas fun was associated with an activity matching and challenging ability. However, it is suggested here that ignoring bitz as an embodied experience, in which an individual is subject to pleasure or pain, or both, risks failing to address the broader implications of participation in or attempting to get into the zone. Indeed activities where transcending into some form of 'other' embodied state (whether or not one wants to call this being in the zone) is an objective for an enhanced performance (or experience) could contribute to situations in which pain becomes normalised or, indeed, overlooked to the detriment of an individual's ultimate wellbeing. Consequently, the notion of moving into a zone and managing pain prompts further questions about whether it is always positive to encourage others to engage in intensive physical activity.

Fun and games

Although the experiences that occurred provide a wealth of material to unpack the complexity of engagement in sport and physical activities, it is, nevertheless, important to take account of some of the, at face value, simple pleasures of movement. Although I have written previously about the importance of fun and enjoyment as a central aspect of participation (Wellard 2013), my experiences during the training did provide further opportunities for me to recognise this,

> It seems like there are lots of activities that are pretty much like adult (or not so adult) versions of childhood play. Things like climbing on bars, skipping, running, jumping, doing handstands and so on.

Although climbing bars and skipping might be considered 'natural' play activities for children, it is interesting to note the extent to which adult bodies are restricted in their movement opportunities. Sport can, therefore, be seen to provide once such space in which adults can have access to playful movements. However, it is not necessarily accessible to everyone (Wellard 2006, 2009) and once 'inside' the forms of play can still be considered highly regulated through adherence to rules and regulations, of not only the specific sport but also the site of the sport (sports club, gym, park, etc.). In addition, and as I mention in my research diary, now that I was starting to get the 'hang of'

CrossFit, the play aspect was becoming more apparent. Getting the 'hang of' CrossFit implies that I had started to master some of the required movements, which meant that participation was becoming easier. In this way, the ability to do an activity significantly impacts on the resulting experience (Evans 2006, Wellard 2006). It is interesting, in an increasingly social media-savvy society that there are many more instances of visual 'evidence' of the will to movement or play by adults that are thwarted by actual ability, or lack of recognition of one's own physical literacy. For example, there are countless clips on the internet of adults (in a bout of playful exuberance) attempting to swing from a rope over a lake or trying to do a high kick on the dance floor, only to misjudge the extent of their weight-bearing capacities or flexibility. Although it is usually the case that when the clips are shown they are intended as a source of amusement, they do also reveal desires to be playful through movement, which often remains dormant. These desires are stored away within a personal memory bank of pleasurable experiences (Wellard 2013), but are nevertheless, not practised or maintained.

Note

1 The McGill Pain Questionnaire is a scale of rating pain developed by Melzack and Torgerson (1971) for medical practitioners. It incorporates a self-report questionnaire that allows individuals to describe the quality and intensity of pain that they are experiencing, most specifically in relation to a medical condition.

6

METAMORPHOSIS

In the summer of 2015 I summarised my thoughts about CrossFit in a simple 'pros and cons' table (see Table 6.1). At the time I wanted to record my feelings before starting the training so that I could reflect upon this at a later stage.

TABLE 6.1 Personal perceptions of CrossFit before starting the training

Appeal	Reservations
1. I get the cross-training aspect. It combines elements of strength training, stamina, flexibility—something that I've always liked doing.	1. I'm not particularly keen on the form that it has adopted in the UK. It seems to be much more ageist and exclusive than the overarching philosophy claims. (I've seen some clubs on the web in the States that do seem to cater for a much broader age/ability group.)
2. I like the intensity of it. You have to take it seriously and you have to commit to it.	2. The intensity of the exercises combined with the way that CrossFit is developing in the UK worries me in that it seems to be unsustainable—in that prolonged participation at such an intensive level suggests that individual engagement might more likely be short term. It seems that a 'go at it hammer and tongs' attitude does not fit in that well with the everyday 'recreational' participant.

3. I like the focus on the individual body and the aspects that allow participation at one's own level—and the opportunity to learn more about one's own body. It allows one to push the body and create challenges.
4. I like the general 'philosophy' of the concept—and this makes the notion of adopting a CrossFit identity appealing.
5. The flexibility of the sessions means that it is easier to fit in when you can—but keep up that affinity/allegiance with the CrossFit 'package'.

3. I am not completely sure about my own ability and whether I will ever be good enough.

On paper, the appeal of CrossFit might seem to outweigh the reservations that I have. However, these reservations might be more significant in the UK—as the opportunities available are much less inclusive. So, although I like the identity (and the theory behind it)—and would probably do so if I could—I do not feel that in the form it is at present it allows me to fit in. I can see the appeal of becoming involved and, in particular, that it might provide the chance to develop a different form of sporting identity. In the past, when someone asked me what sport I did, I would always say a tennis player or swimmer. More recently, I have felt less comfortable saying this as I just don't do these as much—and definitely not at the level I did before. The gym has maybe offered another outlet to continue in some way although I don't see it as an identity, rather something that it allows me to still be active and train in some way. Thus, CrossFit could possibly provide another outlet—as a legitimate identity to engage with and latch on to.

However, while a conventional gym doesn't offer me the same possibilities for a sporting identity in the way that CrossFit does maybe personal training is enough for me.

You're so vain—I bet you think this blog is about you

I don't know if it is just a coincidence, but I have had Carly Simon's song, 'You're so vain', playing in my head recently. Maybe there are some subliminal messages circulating in my mind or that I am becoming aware of a certain form of self-consciousness that could be considered borderline vanity.

There appears to be a definite aspect of vanity or narcissism that prevails in gym-based activities. Whether it is classified in this way is another matter but the focus upon one's own body and constant scrutiny of its 'look', movement and development (in terms of muscularity and weight) does move one in that direction. And while it may not necessarily be the case that all actions are motivated by conscious vanity, many can be read in those terms. For instance, the photo that I placed in my profile was intended as one that would display me in action. However, there was also a degree of editing that reflected a consciousness of the image I wanted to present of myself to an outside world. As such, part of this decision-making process included making sure that the photo did not make me look like Gollum but presented something that represented a legitimate or authentic version of someone taking part in CrossFit.

Subsequently, although there are aspects of my engagement in CrossFit that could be construed as narcissistic, the notion of legitimacy provides an interesting way of thinking about engagement. In this case, I have been aware of the ways in which I have attempted to gain a sense that I am a legitimate participant—or that I do, indeed, 'belong' in some way. My physical performances are the most obvious method to present my body as belonging within this space. However, there are many other things that contribute and part of this is presenting what could be considered a CrossFit identity to the outside world.

More recently I have been aware of my sudden enthusiasm in getting the 'gear' which has meant taking stock of the sports clothing that I have and making assessments about whether it fits the bill for the CrossFit space. I must admit that I have always liked having the latest gear for tennis and the gym. In tennis, as it was a part of my sporting identity, having the latest racquets and sports clothing was an essential aspect of 'being' a tennis player. Similarly, having the 'right' clothing for working out was also important, not only in terms of appropriateness for the activity, but also to convey to others that one had 'knowledge' about training in the gym.

It is, therefore, not surprising that I have done the same as I start to develop a CrossFit identity. 'Getting the gear' is all part of the whole package of an activity such as this, or indeed, any other sport. Nevertheless, this aspect of consumerism is seductive and I hold my hands up and admit to my superficiality in that I have succumbed to it (as I have done before). However, the reason for noting this now is that I want to return to it at a later stage so that I can assess the notion of 'being' legitimate within the CrossFit space and consider the interplay with vanity in terms of how the CrossFit body is (expected to be) presented.

Performance update

The last few months have also been interesting from a social perspective. I said at the start that I was still pretty sceptical about the whole CrossFit 'identity'; however, looking back now, this doesn't seem to have stopped me from embracing it whole-heartedly. Coincidently, last week there were three separate occasions when the topic of 'CrossFitters' came up and it made me think about the extent to which I was actually fitting into the stereotypes that were being discussed. They were as follows:

1. I read an article in a newspaper that was about Christmas office parties and the writer suggested tips for getting through them unscathed. One of the tips was to avoid the 'CrossFit bore', who would manage to bring in CrossFit activities and WoDs [workouts of the day] into every conversation. Upon reading this, I thought about how often I had been bringing in my CrossFit experiences into general conversations and even as examples in some of my lectures.
2. A colleague of mine, who trains at a local gym that also has a CrossFit box attached to it, mentioned how those who attended the box were called 'CrossFit wankers in their nanos' by the regular gym goers. (The nanos are the Reebok shoes that have become de rigueur for CrossFit participants.) It was ironic that I had only just bought a pair the previous week.
3. Even more of a coincidence was when the same colleague sent an email to me with an extract of an interview she had conducted with a gym goer (as part of her research into gym cultures). She thought it would make me laugh as she knew about my training programme. In the conversation the interviewee had remarked upon her observations of the people who took part in CrossFit. According to her, they always seemed to have bigger bags for all their gear. I read this email having just finished my Friday session with coach JP and while I was changing had thought that I needed a bigger bag—so that I could accommodate all of the gear that I was starting to accumulate (knee/wrist/elbow straps, gloves, skipping ropes, protein bars and shakes—clothes, towels, toiletries—training logs, pens)

So maybe, I am embracing a CrossFit identity more than I realise. The intense training programme I have undertaken has undoubtedly meant that it has occupied a substantial part of my everyday life—and because of this I have had to accommodate much of what the 'whole package' of CrossFit requires, in the same way that I would if I were taking on another sport. Nevertheless, there are many aspects that do not necessarily mean I have to 'buy' into the identity so wholeheartedly. That I am doing so suggests the social aspect is appealing to me in the same way that I enjoyed 'presenting' a tennis identity when I played tennis. Even as an older (more hardened) academic, I cannot escape the seductiveness of these performances of sporting capital.

Bipolar CrossFit?

I'm aware that this post is a little bit introspective and may appear somewhat negative. However, with my sociologist hat on, I think it is important to try to understand the feelings of insecurity and doubt that seem to be a constant part of my experiences taking part in a CrossFit training programme. I am attempting to relate these feelings to my previous experiences of training for other sports. For instance, when I trained for tennis matches in my youth, continued practice helped alleviate any doubts I may have harboured about my playing ability and also reassured me that my fitness was at the right level whereas in my training for CrossFit the process is less straightforward and much rockier.

In my very first post I included a table that attempted to outline my feelings about CrossFit before I officially started the training programme. At that stage I had a sense that I was 'on the fence' in that, while I could see a lot of positive benefits for taking part, I also had reservations about the whole CrossFit identity. Although I have attempted to embrace 'doing' CrossFit and maybe in some way I have become part of a CrossFit 'community' I still seem to constantly move from at one moment having an all-embracing feeling of belonging to the next moment having a feeling of being an outsider. These feelings manifest themselves in a range of ways.

While these bipolar feelings of (CrossFit) worth may be considered predominantly psychological, the physical aspects undoubtedly contribute to how I interpret them. Sometimes, at the end of a session, one where I feel I have given 100% in terms of physical effort and concentration, I do feel that I warrant some form of recognition or identification as a legitimate CrossFit 'athlete'. There is a sense of satisfaction and almost a belief that because I have given so much of myself, physically and mentally, it is an indication of belonging. At the same time, awareness that I am developing more knowledge about techniques, terminology and 'how to do' CrossFit indicates to me that I am in some ways a bone fide CrossFitter. Nevertheless, these feelings of belonging are unstable. It seems to me that when I am away from the gym and not actually doing it the feelings of insecurity about a CrossFit identity become more apparent. Much of these feelings of being an outsider are fuelled by the general messages presented either on YouTube or on the CrossFit games website—where the general portrayal of a 'typical' CrossFit participant is either youthful or a former weightlifter or bodybuilder. There appears to be a constant tension between the general mantra of inclusivity and that anybody can do CrossFit, whereas the reality (like so many fitness-related gyms) is that the projected ideal is very much based upon a particular type of youthful and excessively muscular body.

Like in other sports and predominantly in the media these elite ideal types are presented as role models to be aspired to. However, the ultimate effect is more likely to be the reverse in that they create a sense of unrealistic goals. For example, it is a major part of CrossFit (and in general most sports) that progress is monitored through recording personal bests. Thus, in the case of my training programme (and as I mentioned in my last post about progress) recording a maximum weight, say on the deadlift, provides a useful way to establish benchmarks one sets as targets. This is all well and good and does provide a sense of achievement, particularly when it becomes clear that one can lift a heavier weight than previously. So, when the other week we were working on deadlifts to explore what my current maximum rep for this was, I managed to get to 100 kg. Putting this in context, especially in terms of what I could actually lift at the start of last year, being able to do this was a considerable achievement and there was a sense of satisfaction at accomplishing this weight. However, constantly in the back of my mind was an awareness of what 'others' were doing. In this case, those others were the ones that were appearing on YouTube and doing lifts of 250 kg. Consequently, evaluations of my performance were made bearing in mind the performances of others with the effect that (for me) my weaknesses were highlighted, and, subsequently, fuelled further negative feelings that I was not making the grade. Even putting things in further context (factors such as my age, weight [64 kg] and relative newness to CrossFit) do not necessarily dispel the feelings of not being 'good enough' and, ultimately, not being a proper or 'authentic' CrossFitter.

Why I should worry about this and make it such an issue is a good question. I am not sure when I entered into this research that 'becoming' a CrossFitter was something that I had wanted to do. However, as I have mentioned in other posts, the process of taking part has meant that negotiating a particular identity is a core aspect of participation. Reflecting upon all of this is useful in that it helps me get to the heart of why I am doing all of this. While the period that I have allocated to conducting this research is drawing to an end, I know that

I will continue to 'do' CrossFit. Whether how I actually do practice it corresponds with the format prescribed within what is becoming a 'traditional' CrossFit box does not really matter. What is important is that I have also recognised that my prime objective is to maintain a passion for 'doing' physical activity and exercise in ways that my body can.

Metamorphosis complete?

Metamorphosis is a great word. It was a word that came into my head yesterday when I had an email from CrossFit.com telling me that I had successfully passed my level 1 CrossFit trainer course. The news coincided with the completion of my six-month period of training and made me take stock of my relatively short CrossFit journey. It is now approaching the end of February and I am on a rest week prior to the announcement of the qualifying events for the 2016 CrossFit Games tomorrow. This means that I have now achieved what I set out to do when I first started in September last year. This was to complete (or get through) the training programme and register for the Games. At that time I hadn't really thought too much about transformations, but it is only now that I can see how much I have metamorphosed into some form of CrossFit creature.

In Kafka's (2007) *Metamorphosis* the central character, Gregor, turns into an unidentified insect-like creature that he finds repellent and so too do the people he comes into contact with. Hopefully, that

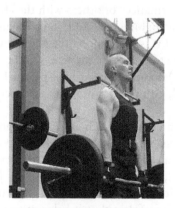 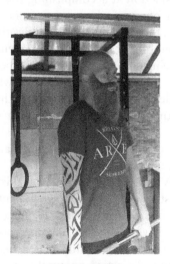

September 2015   February 2016

FIGURES 6.1 Before and after training

is not what has happened in my case. I'm using the analogy with meta-morphosis in terms of the notion of transformation and rather than this being a process that just happens there is much more input by the individual through learning, experience and 'performance'. So, in the case of my initial intentions to undergo a period of CrossFit training so that I could be exposed to a range of embodied experiences, this process has revealed far more about questions of identity and performance than I had initially expected. I hadn't at that time been completely aware of the many other 'requirements' of becoming a CrossFit athlete. Although, in my first post, I had outlined some of my reservations about what CrossFit represented and whether I would be able to fit in, these were concerned more with my own perceptions of my ability. However, it is interesting to reflect, now that I have completed the six months, how other boxes have been ticked along the way—boxes which appear to present a checklist for what a CrossFit participant should tick off (and, indeed, look like).

Although my original goal was to complete the whole period of six months' training, in addition I have now registered for the CrossFit games and last weekend I attended a level 1 training course which means now, according to the email that I received, I am a level 1 CrossFit trainer. Although this is not necessarily very remarkable it is interesting on many other levels, especially when I think that this time last year I wasn't really completely sure about what CrossFit was. Now, according to this certificate, I have become legitimate within the world of CrossFit. Thinking about it from this perspective makes me realise that there has been a transformation of some kind and although I do like the idea that I've biologically turned into some other form of creature in the way that Kafka describes, it is nevertheless interesting to think about transformation in terms of the social and temporal aspects. I'm using the Kafka analogy purposely because it is dramatic but also to demonstrate the seemingly bizarre aspects of social and individual constructions of identity. Negotiating and manoeuvring through my relationship with a CrossFit identity has ended up preoc-cupying me throughout the past six months much more than my initial

TABLE 6.2 CrossFit checklist

Suffer numerous injuries	☐
Attend CrossFit box	☐
Buy lots of CrossFit gear	☐
Take part in the CrossFit Games	☐
Take level 1 CrossFit trainer course	☐
Get tattoos	☐ (?)
(For males) grow beard	☐ (?)

fears about my physical capabilities and my capacity to cope with the physical demands of the activities.

So, now that I have had this new identity bestowed upon me, rather than feeling like Gregor in *Metamorphosis* maybe I should really feel like the scarecrow in the *Wizard of Oz*. When he received his certificate from the wizard it provided 'proof' to the world that he was intelligent and he subsequently 'became' intelligent. That might apply to the scarecrow, but in my case I am not so convinced about my CrossFit credentials on the basis of my certificate. I still have so many causes for doubt and maybe there are a couple of significant ones remaining. . . .

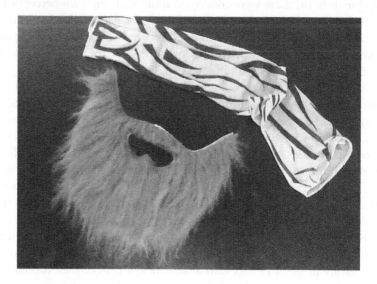

FIGURE 6.2 Beard and tattoo

7

IDENTITIES AND POWER

I'm in control?

Guess what? I now have a beard! At the end of the last chapter I said (albeit light-heartedly) that there were two things that cast doubts about my legitimacy as a bona fide CrossFitter—getting tattoos and growing a beard. However, during the summer of 2016, after completing the training and then taking part in the CrossFit Open and gaining some CrossFit coaching qualifications, the temptation was too great and I thought I would experiment with growing a beard. I had never had one previously in my life and in the early stages of training I felt a little too self-conscious to actually grow one because it felt like a step too far and a little too obvious. I do not really know if there was a specific moment when I made the decision, although it seemed like a 'natural' process. Thinking about this now, although growing a beard seems like such a trivial aspect of the whole process of engaging with CrossFit, there are many things that it reveals about social identity formation and my active participation within it. Not only is this in terms of the explicit symbolic meaning that a beard might convey, but also there is an extent to which I was complicit in the way that I performed the obvious symbols of expressing a particular identity. Subsequently, I conformed to the (socially generated) expectations of what being a CrossFit athlete should entail and 'look like'. These aspects of my complicity, whether intentional or unintentional, need to be explored further and it is in this chapter that I want to unpack, through the example of my own 'metamorphosis', questions relating to embodied control, complicity and compliance.

Janet Jackson informs us in her song 'I'm in control' that she is now in a situation where she has taken charge. This declaration is very much a statement of the times in that we try to convince ourselves (and more importantly others) that we are in charge of our destinies. It fits in quite nicely with the neo-liberal mantra of empowerment, which asserts that everyone has the opportunity to achieve what they want and be successful—and in doing so should not let anyone get in their way or dictate what they should do.

Even if this were possible, I am not really convinced that the implications for a society of self-obsessed and mercenary individuals would be that appealing or would have really been thought through in any rational way—that is, apart from those marketing executives who create the seductive images of fiercely independent and successful individuals, in the hope of lucrative financial gain from the products they are promoting.

Although the need to be in control can be interpreted in a range of ways, it remains, nevertheless, seductive. Consequently, it does take a lot of convincing to acknowledge that one really is not at all in control but is rather left at the mercy of serendipitous forces (as well as marketing executives), which are constantly generating knowledge that endorses the message that one is able to do exactly as one wants to do (that is, if they work hard to achieve it).

Although the metamorphosis that I describe in Chapter 6 may draw on some elements of artistic licence, the intention was to convey the notion of identity movement. The comparison was provided as a mechanism to highlight that the 'transformation' encompassed both social and physiological changes, changes that were not only experienced by myself but also recognised and influenced by others. By maintaining a research diary throughout the process, I was able to look back at the entries and attempt to build a picture of this embodied transition. It was, indeed, one of the most unexpected aspects of this process, and it is only now that I can 'stand back' and attempt to interpret what happened throughout this period.

In the two years since I started the training programme, it has become apparent that I am now known as 'Ian who does CrossFit' by my colleagues in my department. Here, CrossFit is now coterminous with 'Ian' and appears to dictate the way in which social interactions are staged—not only with colleagues who engage in CrossFit, but also with others who do not have any background knowledge about what CrossFit entails, apart from awareness that it incorporates some form of fitness training. In the same way that prior knowledge that someone is, for instance, a keen football enthusiast shapes the direction of opening conversations, so does prior knowledge that I am a CrossFit enthusiast provide the context in which conversations develop. This transformation in the way that I am now perceived is noticeable because I have been known to my colleagues and a member of the department for many years before my participation in it and I cannot remember being aware of any association with a specific identity, other than that of my academic role.

At this stage, it is worth highlighting one of the points I made in the research diary as it forms the central message in this chapter:

> I am not sure that when I entered into this research 'becoming' a CrossFitter was something that I had wanted to do. However, as I have mentioned in other posts, the process of taking part has meant that negotiating a particular identity is a core aspect of participation. Reflecting upon all of this is useful in that it helps me get to the heart of why I am doing all of this.

To an extent, the process of recording my experiences provided a mechanism to 'stand back' from myself. Although this is something that we all do in various forms, the diary and photos become a form of evidence that I can reflect upon along with my memories. In this way, I can attempt to look at myself not necessarily in a detached manner but with a degree of distance that enables me to explain these experiences within a social context. Consequently, what follows is further exploration into the embodied aspects that have been significant, with which I have engaged either intentionally or unintentionally. More specifically, these are the themes that dominate Chapter 6 that relate to the signs and symbols of identity presentation, complicity and control.

Signs and symbols

Although it may appear relatively insignificant, the beard offers a significant symbol in terms of the transformation that I talk about. It reminds me of Barthes' (1977) description of cultural signs that signify, in obvious ways, meaning. This was especially the case for Barthes in popular culture, notably visual media such as film, television and advertising. Although there has been criticism of his generalisations within academic circles (for instance, Sobchack 2004), the symbols that Barthes describes are, nevertheless, apparent to the general audience who recognise these (obvious) symbols with an awareness that they denote exaggerated cultural characteristics. It is possible that the critics of Barthes display a mild contempt for the mass audience in that they make assumptions about the viewer's ability to distinguish how these signs are being presented. The process of engaging with a visual form such as a film necessitates a level of awareness in the process and a sense of complicity in allowing forms of manipulation, and any subsequent exaggeration of the signs (like a pantomime) is recognised as part of the experience.

More recent mass expansion of the media in its various forms has increased the need for instantly recognisable signs, particularly for those involved in advertising and image making. The extent to which the viewer knowingly enters into these interactions is a discussion that will continue to trouble academics in cultural studies. However, although these debates about media representation and audience engagement are not the focus of this book, the questions that emerge in terms of agency and complicity remain relevant to my exploration of embodied experience in sport and physical activity. Signs and symbols of sporting identity adopt similar patterns. The 'mythologies' that Barthes describes are equally apparent in sporting contexts (Whannel & Wellard 1995, Whannel 2006). Mythologies are therefore what Barthes was implying, i.e. culturally determined creations. In this way, we can understand how instant (universally recognised) connections become even more attractive in an increasingly divergent and complex global society.

The rise of a global consumer culture is important to acknowledge if we are attempting to understand representations of the body, in terms of not only the visual representation but also the ways in which this broader knowledge is internalised and acted on. Featherstone (2010) looks at the relationship between the body and the image of the body (in terms of the way that the individual and society see the body) within the context of a consumer society. Here, he shows how body image is generally understood in terms of an object that is seen by others and is a direct representation of the self or that person. He relates this to the general inference of physiognomy, where there is an assumption that the body and, more specifically, the face are reflections of the self and character. In this way, the beard that I have talked about provides an obvious object that represents specific (socio-historical) cultural characteristics.

Featherstone explores this further by highlighting the ways in which understandings of transformation have become important, particularly in the areas of body modification and addressing the outward look of the body. In doing so, he suggests that society has developed a simplistic logic which is both understood by the individual and ultimately exploited by a consumer culture that sells products that can be understood as accessories or aids to achieving a transformation of the self.

Featherstone highlights the need to recognise the broader dimensions of body image and understandings of the body through acknowledgment of body schema, which is a non-visual sense of the body and, indeed, ventures towards the notion of embodiment.

Featherstone does this by acknowledging the importance of synaesthesia, or the way in which the sensors work together to produce not only our perception of the world, but the way we sense other bodies when we encounter them in everyday life. Drawing upon Taussig's (1991) notion of the tactile eye, Featherstone suggests the following:

> The senses in movement can be seen as closely related to affect. Other bodies and the images of other bodies in the media and consumer culture may literally move us, make us feel moved, by affecting our bodies in inchoate ways that cannot easily be assimilated to conceptual thought. Here we think of the shiver down the spine or the gut feeling. Affect points to the experience of intensities, to the way in which media images are felt through bodies. This applies to bodies in motion, or imbued with the possibility of movement, as opposed to the type of ocular narcissistic identification we get with the mirror-image of a static unified body-and-face.
>
> *(Featherstone 2010, p. 195)*

It is important to account for the senses and the way that they affect our interpretation of the signs of consumer culture—signs that are both manipulative and seductive, which we can 'buy into' and then employ as mechanisms to present an identity that projects us beyond the everyday person. Consequently, it is worth attempting to explore the processes through which we seek to 'distinguish' ourselves from others. Although I have drawn on the theories of Foucault in previous chapters to explain the arbitrary and completing forms of knowledge, within the context of contemporary consumer culture it seems only relevant to acknowledge the prevalence of social knowledge which celebrates the notion of distinguishing oneself from another. I am specifically referring here to Bourdieu's (1986) concept of distinction, which was grounded in a critique of the hierarchical structure of society, dominated by economic and class disparity. Although I am aware of the conflicting trajectories from which Foucault and Bourdieu developed their ideas, it is difficult to ignore the dominance of class and economic factors that operate within contemporary western society and the influence that capitalism has on twenty-first century knowledge. Although I adopt a broader embodied approach to my thinking, it is nevertheless important to consider the influence of economic factors and the way that they drive neoliberal and neoconservative frameworks, which in turn drive mainstream political thought (Rose 1999, Phipps 2014)

For Bourdieu, power is expressed through the ability of those (who have access to power) to define what society holds in distinction. Unlike Marx, it was no longer the means of production that constituted domination, but socially recognised taste that has the capacity to determine terms of distinction. Domination is reproduced and mediated by knowledge and expression of 'taste'. Thus, for Bourdieu, the social system within which knowledge is generated or dispositions are organised (which he described as the 'habitus') reflects a member's internalisation, as natural, of the taste of their class.

In terms of establishing a class position, habitus often involves the social presentation of taste as natural or 'second nature'. The notion of second nature is a predominant feature in body presentation. For example, in contemporary society, greater esteem is given to those who are able to present social performances of 'natural beauty'. An individual who has achieved a specific body image through, for instance, excessive training, dieting, steroids or plastic surgery does not carry the same cultural capital as a slender model who can eat anything without gaining weight or the handsome actor born with a good 'bone structure'.

Bourdieu's ideas are also relevant in that he describes the social world and the way individuals achieve understanding of this social world through bodily practice. The concept of practice is particularly relevant because it provides a means of acknowledging the role of the individual and individual experience in wider social relations. For Bourdieu, practice is first located in space and in time and, second, it is not consciously organised and orchestrated. For instance, Bourdieu talks about social relations in terms of how an individual develops:

> 'a feel for the game' through, 'a mastery acquired by experience of the game, and one which works outside of conscious control and discourse (in a way that, for instance, techniques of the body do) . . .'
>
> *(Bourdieu 1990, p. 61)*

Bourdieu's concept of a social actor learning the rules of the game draws on an interpretation of doxic experience that relates to the notion that people take themselves and their social world for granted. In doing so, they do not think about it because they do not have to. Consequently, developing knowledge about market practices is considered an everyday aspect of social knowledge, and becoming consumer 'savvy' is taken for granted as a skill that needs to be developed as a participant in an increasingly competitive market place.

Bourdieu's metaphor of social life as a game does have problems, however, as Jenkins (1992) points out. Games have rules and are learnt through explicit teaching as well as practice, which is important for social competence. However, in sport, excellence is prioritised whereas only competence is needed for the habitus. The problem with this description is that Bourdieu does not fully account for the difference between competence and excellence. This is a factor particularly in the sports field where competence allows participation, but only to an extent. Social constructions, such as gender and sexuality, create barriers to participation regardless of competence or excellence. Thus, within sport, the continued focus on excellence, in the form of idealised versions of bodily performance, is not fully covered by the concepts of taste and cultural capital when taking into account gender and sexuality.

An important aspect of this relates to Hexus, which can be considered to form the style and manner in which actors perform, such as gait, stance or gesture. Hexus presents a social performance of where the individual is located within the habitus. It also demonstrates the importance of the body in Bourdieu's conceptualisation of the habitus. Through bodily hexis the idiosyncratic (the personal) combines with the systematic (the social) and mediates a link between an individual's subjective world and the cultural world into which he or she is born and which she or he shares with others. Thus, the body can be seen as a device through which cultural signs are imprinted and internalised through a socialisation and learning process. Importantly, as Jenkins notes, 'the habitus is inculcated as much, if not more, by experience as by explicit teaching' (Jenkins 1992, p. 76).

In habitus, power derives from the taken-for-granted aspects of the performances. Socially competent performances are produced through routine, in the sense that the actor's competence is demonstrated by them not necessarily knowing what they are doing. Thus, in my experiences of being socialised into CrossFit culture, in my eagerness to embrace what it was I needed to do to participate effectively, I did not really have the wherewithal to reflect critically on my actions at the time.

Although it may seem that, within the context of sport and physical activity, movement is an obvious prerequisite, there is still a range of 'static' symbols that present knowledge about what is being presented, and these ultimately affect the way in which both the presenter and the viewer respond to the symbol. In CrossFit it might be argued that there is a greater requirement for participants to be seen to be active and able to perform their CrossFit credentials through displays of physical activity. Here, the body is foregrounded and offered as a sign of both a CrossFit identity and physical capital through demonstrations of strength, fitness and muscularity, and implied strength and fitness through recognisable signs of being a CrossFitter. There are similarities to the way in which the conventional sporting body is presented and understood within contemporary society, but the CrossFitter's body might be considered even more so, in a similar way to the personal trainer's body, described in Chapter 3.

Bearing in mind the relevance of the 'signs' that operate within certain contexts as described above, in this case the CrossFit community, it is worth considering the factors that shaped the process of my CrossFit identity formation and the specific ways that it occurred during my participation. These might be described as follows:

a. *Language of CrossFit*

CrossFit, like any other 'club', generates a system of implicit and explicit rules of engagement. Consequently, one important aspect of the 'whole package' (Wellard 2013) of CrossFit is acquiring appropriate knowledge and being able to display language that is specific to it. However, as well as learning the terminology that has been created to describe distinct CrossFit movements and activities (such as WoDs [workouts of the day]/AMRAPs [as many rounds as possible]/EMOMs [every minute on the minute]/ girls) there were also terms that have been incorporated from existing sports, such as weightlifting and gymnastics (for example, cleans, jerks, planks and muscle-ups). Consequently, my research reflected that it was overwhelming, at the start, attempting to gain a sufficient grasp of the extensive language—that was considered essential to take part successfully. Indeed, when I attended different CrossFit boxes, I noticed that there was an expectation that participants would be aware of the terminology.

b. *Presenting a CrossFit appearance through accessories*

I mentioned in Chapter 6 how a colleague had made disparaging remarks about the CrossFit participants who trained at the gym she attended. This particular CrossFit area was attached to the regular gym and those taking part in CrossFit sessions had to walk through the main gym to get to it. The 'CrossFit wankers' were mainly identified through their appearance, which was distinct from the regular gym goers. Specific CrossFit attire was crucial in marking out these distinctions. Reebok- or Rogue-branded clothing was considered de rigueur and the manufacturers had latched on to the appeal among CrossFit participants that clothing would provide one way to separate them from regular gym trainers. There were also accessories that were essential for many of the activities, such as knee sleeves, elbow sleeves, wrist straps and long socks used to protect the shins during deadlifts and cleans). These and many others contributed to the comment about CrossFit participants having bigger bags than the gym goers.

c. *Appearance through the body*

I have mentioned the profusion of beards among male CrossFit athletes but there were also other ways that the body presented confirmation to others of 'being' a legitimate CrossFitter. Muscularity (for both men and women) was an obvious outcome of engaging in hard training. Although this has been evident in other forms of gym and bodybuilding training, a particular form of physical body was noticeable. For the majority of both men and women, showing off defined abdomens and general 'ripped' bodies was considered acceptable in the box. Men could perform the workouts without shirts, whereas the women could wear sports bras. However, gender distinctions were made through conventional displays of beards for the men and long hair for women.

Not only were bodies central in displaying the effects of the physical training, but also there were associated movements that could be seen as being both an outcome of the physical transformations in the body and more contrived in terms of how the body moved. For example, the variety of movements experienced in CrossFit can be seen to shape the particular forms of bodily hexis that Bourdieu describes. Although excessive participation in body building can lead to a 'bodybuilder's walk' (Fussell 1992), as a result of overdeveloped muscles (such as quadriceps and latissimus dorsi) which contribute to a form of waddling gait, in CrossFit focus on other movements means excessive muscular definition can be seen to impede performance. Consequently, the influence of movements from gymnastics and weightlifting, which focus on maintaining the core and moving with weights, as well as cardiovascular activities, shapes a body that can be seen to move and present itself in a different way.

d. *Performance of specific CrossFit movements*

Relating to the previous point, as well as the requirement for knowledge of the language of CrossFit, there was also the expectation that one would eventually be able to perform specific movements and demonstrate knowledge through the body of specific technique required for movements, such as the clean and jerk or pull-up. In this way knowledge could be seen (and kudos achieved) through demonstrations of technique—and being able to perform movements that were considered beyond the ability of regular gym goers. These included muscle-ups, double-unders, pull ups and ring dips, as well as traditional Olympic weightlifting movements.

Complicity

Having started to acquire the 'knowledge' described above, I made a conscious effort to present as what I considered a CrossFit athlete should look like. I started to do this after only a few months into the training. I wanted to present an image that I had formulated about CrossFit and present this to others. My initial justification was very much related to making an obvious display as a means of confronting what I considered to be an ageist perception of sport. My rationale was that I would provide evidence that an older person can do a physically challenging activity like CrossFit. Although my hope was that people would look approvingly at the way I had embraced CrossFit and recognise it as an indication that it was ok for older people to still participate in vigorous sport, I was still aware (and willing to acknowledge) that many might think 'who is that silly old fool' or something even more disparaging, along the lines of 'mutton dressed as lamb'. Nevertheless, I convinced myself that I was taking a stand.

Although my rationale for making a political statement about ageist discrimination may have provided a worthwhile (and academically legitimate) central element for my embracing of all things CrossFit, I cannot ignore what might be considered the more 'uncomfortable truths' in my willingness to embrace it so wholeheartedly. The fact that I could do it in the first place meant that I possessed sporting capital from the onset. It was not like I was starting something from scratch because I have always been reasonably fit, and my abilities transferred to many of the core CrossFit activities. Even though I had many weaknesses in relation to some of the movements, these were not to the extent that I could not develop further. That I could achieve the basic levels of fitness required to participate was a bonus and galvanised my subsequent enthusiasm to continue.

My location in a sports department was also a contributing factor. CrossFit provided further evidence to staff and students that I was a 'legitimate' member of a sporting community. I had something to replace the 'I do tennis' badge that I was aware was becoming less evident and increasingly something that I 'used to do'.

The feelings of self-worth related to being able to 'still do it' were a major consideration in my continued participation. Wearing the T-shirt was a sign for me as well as to others that I was still 'productive' and could contribute in some way. In other words, my body, along with the accessories, provided an opportunity for me to declare that:

I am still an active man—a sportsman

The notion of me being complicit also raises the question about the extent to which I am in fact reinforcing the stereotypes of old age. Training for and taking part in the CrossFit Open 'distinguished' me (in the Bourdieusian sense) from other men of my age. Completing all the events at RX signalled not only to myself, but also to others that I was more physically able than most men my age.

Therefore, although these may fuel my own sense of self-worth and vanity, there are other ways that my actions might be perceived. By attempting to convince others that I was not 'old' in the conventional sense, it could be argued that I was trying to disassociate myself from other older people and, in doing so, could be reinforcing a young/old binary, in a similar way to what Butler (1993) describes as occurring in the reiteration of gender binaries. Although I am aware of these tensions it is still, nevertheless, difficult to fully separate my egotistical agenda from the research practice. My reaction to conventional perceptions of ageing might, on one the hand, be considered as a form of individual empowered action, but, on the other, my actions could also be seen as 'othering' or distancing, particularly if my actions are not seen as representative, or I am considered a freak of old age.

I mention this, as I became increasingly aware of 'age', as a factor that I felt more conscious about compared with other forms of exclusion that I have explored previously, such as ability or sexuality (Wellard 2002, 2006). Consequently, my research radar became more sensitive to situations where I felt that age was an issue. However, there were different ways in which I sought to negotiate these tensions. Although I attempted to maintain a research agenda that accommodated an inclusive approach, egoistical elements that contributed to my embodied identity might not have always readily assisted how successful I was in achieving this aim. I can relate this to previous research where, once again, conflicting agendas managed to compete during the research process. When gathering the data for my research into sporting masculinities (Wellard 2009) there were similar embodied conflicts of interest. In this case, the focus of the research was on how the body was central to performances of masculinity in sport contexts. Here, my agenda was based on challenging the domination of heteronormative masculine practices in traditional sports at the expense of subordinated masculinities, where I had positioned myself as a 'representative' of sporting masculinity that could be inclusive. During one encounter, before an interview, I had arranged to play a singles match (in tennis) with the prospective interviewee. Playing tennis (whether a game or coaching session) was a strategy I had incorporated into other interviews in the hope that, by taking part in an activity that was mutually enjoyable, it would help provide a suitable 'warm-up' before an interview. However, the subsequent match on this occasion became extremely competitive and over-heated. In this situation, my sporting ego took over and, rather than thinking about the interview that followed, I became determined to win. The following is an extract from my research diary.

It was obvious that Tim was really annoyed about losing and found it hard to say anything when we had finished. I could not say to him that I had not really been concentrating initially, but also did not want to be patronising and say that he had played well. At the same time I thought that it would be difficult to conduct an interview and suggested that we did it some other time. I was disappointed with myself, for letting the situation become so competitive and losing perspective of the social situation. However, the example highlights a number of factors. In this particular situation I was involved in the social process of performing expected sporting masculinity and, at that moment, complying with broader hegemonic masculine practices. Although we were gay men and aware of the social discrimination which takes place at the expense of alternative sexuality, within the arena of sport we succumbed to the prevailing expected sporting masculine sensibilities which diverted our attention from the original social setting both of us had entered. In this particular case, the practices prevalent in mainstream sport overshadowed the more egalitarian sensibilities which might have been expected to be displayed within the context of the gay and lesbian movement. To that extent, Tim and I conformed more to the mainstream version of sport rather than confronted it. The cultural significance of sport brings with it the knowledge that there is capital to be gained from taking part or being able to display evidence of this. Often, the awareness of being gay and occupying subordinate sexuality is displaced by the need to present expected sporting masculinity. This is further exaggerated by the perception that gay men should attempt to be as good as 'real' men. Consequently, these performances reinforce discriminatory gender practices rather than confront them.

(Wellard 2009, p. 63)

I have included the above extract because there is a similarity with the form of intentionality that might have been operating during this research. Specifically, throughout the period that I have been engaging in CrossFit, and just like my experiences researching men taking part in sport, I cannot ignore my initial motivations for exploring these areas and assume that any academic training I have received will automatically provide immunity from the prevailing discourses of sport and age. Although it was apparent that discourses of hegemonic masculinity, operating in sporting contexts, influenced the way that I reacted to the sporting contest described above, it is not unreasonable to suggest that these might emerge in other sporting contexts.

Consequently, it is not unreasonable to suggest that the 'chip on my shoulder' relating to performances of sporting masculinity that I harboured in previous research has not been removed entirely.

Uncomfortable truths

As much I would like to think that I can conduct my research with an invisible shield that protects me from bias and prejudice, I am susceptible to the weaknesses of my own humanity and the darker (market) forces that operate within a capitalist system which juxtaposes exploitation with 'profit' and success. Just like Frodo in Tolkien's *Lord of the Rings* (1992), the lure of the (neo-liberal) ring is compelling and can cloud one's initial integrity. However, rather than keep the ring on or enter into some Faustian pact with the devil where there is no going back, reflecting upon and being open to the potential frailties of one's own ego is a mechanism to keep 'things in check'.

This form of reflexive self-analysis is helpful in relation to exploring the initial assumptions and motivations for doing the research in the first place. For instance, there are times when the tensions mentioned above are not just entirely related to CrossFit but can be readily associated with sport in general, in that there remains a conflict of interest—in terms of the drive for performance (which promotes an inward form of self-interested determination)—and that of community cohesion and inclusion. For it is the embodied self that is informed by a barrage of competing forms of knowledge, affecting the physical, social and psychological facets of being—to varying degrees in different social spaces. For example, I have described previously why I enjoy going to the gym:

> As I have aged, I have realised that I enjoy working out at the gym more. A significant factor in this assessment is my awareness that I am less conscious of comparing myself to other men or other bodies in the way I was during my twenties. However, there are still elements of vanity that influence my motivations for participation. I am conscious that I do not want to look like a 'typical' middle-aged man with a large belly. I want to be lithe and flexible in a way that makes me not want to take up too much space or attract attention. There are a number of competing sensibilities here. They relate to my perceptions of power relations, sexuality and heteronormativity. I realise that these are conflicting discourses which are operating within the context of heterosexuality and gay masculinity.
>
> *(Wellard 2013, p. 117)*

Although this reflection was written only a few years ago, if I take into consideration my recent experiences participating in CrossFit as part of the research described in this book, I can see that I need to reconsider those thoughts. The reflections above suggest that the way in which I was engaging in gym training was more 'controlled', possibly because of the way that I was engaging with it. In this case, it was as an 'invisible', independent participant engaging in a large, commercial, global gym. The appeal was in my ability to be anonymous and I found that my older body was also one that was more likely to be ignored. The contrast was even more evident because of my previous experience playing tennis and having established an identity that (I felt) necessitated displays of sporting ability. However, a CrossFit identity expects (or demands) more outward displays of ability and achievement. This was evident not only throughout the training programme where there was a sense of obligation in my relationship with my coach in terms of the shared goal, but also in the general mantra relating to taking part in and 'belonging to' a CrossFit community.

However, there are other sentiments that remain salient. My attempts at maintaining a slim, active body continues to appeal to my efforts to resist both the social stereotypes of old age and that of the older (heteronormative) *male*. Here, it is not just an attempt to slow down the impending decrepitude of old age, but also to avert (through bodily presentation) unwanted recognition that I might be presenting a certain 'type' of masculinity. Just like the signs that Barthes describes (mentioned above), the excesses of the corporate, middle-aged man can be seen to be symbolised through embodied signs, such as the wide girth and grey suit.

The appeal of CrossFit could thus be considered as a counterfoil to such a representation. Although CrossFit claims to have been established as an alternative to the extensive, commercial practices of global gyms, it is in the general outward presentation of a CrossFit participant often similar to that of the 'hipster or maverick, who provides evidence of the rejection of the trappings of corporate living (Murphy 2012). Nevertheless, these claims are contested (Dawson 2017) and, although the initial boxes that emerged in garages and backyards might support alternative philosophical and political statements, more recent developments in CrossFit suggest that it is evolving into an equally global commercial behemoth

Irrespective of the general perception of CrossFit, my body does provide the opportunity to display a sign of alternativity or even alterity—particularly in terms of stereotypes of the older male body and class.

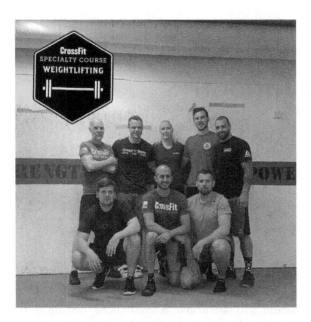

FIGURE 7.1 Part of the community? (Ian, far left back row)

8

FINAL THOUGHTS

Without meaning to sound like a tired cliché, getting to the stage of gathering together these final thoughts for this book has occurred only after what could be considered a *journey*, albeit a tortuous journey. My experiences have been not only about enduring the physical training, but also more about negotiating a pathway that has taken me further outside of my academic comfort zones.

In previous writing, much of the process of finding ways to respond to and address a research question was based on more conventional approaches where I would set out to gather information from either other people or secondary sources. The data I collected would then provide the focus for subsequent analysis and writing. This would usually involve editing vast amounts of material so that a reasonable abridged picture of the research could be presented to the reader. Although I attempted to incorporate a reflexive approach in my research, and did incorporate aspects of my own experiences as a mechanism to generate questions and guide my analysis, the final versions of work that I produced still managed to keep me at a distance.

In more recent years, however, I have realised that reflection and contemplation of personal experiences can provide an effective way to account for the complexity of embodied practices. Often it is the case, in many qualitative sociological research studies, that claims for incorporating inductive approaches do not necessarily avoid the influence of deduction. It could even be suggested that it is considered an easier option to venture out into the field, armed with a series of predetermined questions (or remain at one's desk and use modern technology) with no other intention than to find out what one hoped to in the first place. In all of this, there remains an expectation to deliver a nicely packaged research project that offers some semblance of a conclusion. The trouble is life is not like that and it is difficult (nigh impossible) to neatly sum up aspects of a social world that are generally complex.

Consequently, the overall aim of a book that set out to explore the question of 'whose body is it anyway' was never going to reach a tidy conclusion. But recognising this in the first place made it easier to remain open to ideas that would or could emerge during the process of engaging in an embodied practice, such as physical fitness training. Indeed, the decision to allow myself to participate in the process, rather than explore the experiences of others undergoing similar training, was productive in a range of ways that might not have emerged (if at all) in more conventional (and possibly safer) forms of research.

Much of the raison d'être for this book has been to demonstrate how qualitative research can be meaningful, especially within the context of exploring embodied experience. Where many studies that claim to adopt qualitative principles fail is when they engage in what Hammersley and Atkinson (1995, p. 21) describe as 'futile appeals to empiricism'. In many cases the interpretation of material collected incorporates approaches more suited to quantitative forms of measurement and attempts to achieve an impression of objectivity. Rather than explore and elaborate on ideas that emerge during the research, there appears to remain an unnecessary expectation to provide generalisations and forms of quantification, regardless of the subjectivity apparent in the initial research question.

Uncomfortable research

The notion of complicity, described in Chapter 7, not only resonates with the methodological issues mentioned above, but also, by association, has an implication for any subsequent theoretical claims made. Self-reflexivity, although essential in any attempts to address the problems faced with conducting research, is, nevertheless, difficult precisely because it makes the researcher sometimes confront uncomfortable personal 'truths', truths that can be hidden in most forms of conventional research.

Although a quest for truth represents what might be considered the motive for most research, just like the discussion of wellbeing in Chapter 3, it is hard to pinpoint what it should look like. I am reminded of a colleague who would often start a sentence with 'to be honest', which always made me wonder, if he needed to make such a declaration in the first place, what it meant when he did not start with it? The point here is that making a claim to be honest or truthful suggests that one is making distinctions between a statement that is considered true based on some form of comparison and other statements that are considered untruthful or, indeed, false. By adopting an approach where one sets the scene by making a claim that one is being honest on a specific occasion, but not on others, there is the suggestion that there are a range of 'truths' or levels of truthfulness, determined subjectively by the individual making such declarations. If this is the case, then attempts to find truth and, ultimately, seek objectivity are meaningless, unless they are acknowledged and elaborated on in relation to the subjective account.

Much of the process of exploring any question is to reflect upon and unpack where the interest (or the motivation to do the research) has been generated in the first place. This is a quality that is generally encouraged in most aspects of postgraduate research. However, it is more often the case that any realisation of interest recognised by the researcher is at the same time systematically 'discouraged' through subsequent engagement with academic practices, and has an emphasis to be seen to adopt scientific methods. Although the 'interest' displayed by the researcher at the onset of a research project is generally influenced by their own personal biography, contemporary discourses of knowledge and, possibly, areas of research that fit into a current academic zeitgeist are equally significant. What I am suggesting here is that there is often little consideration for the impact of the initial orientation and disposition of the researcher on the possible pathway that the research might take. This is important in the subsequent development of a nuanced train of thought and, specifically, any theoretical claims made.

Reflexivity enables more detailed unpacking of the underlying meaning of social experience—in other words life experience. By recognising that exploring one's own lived experiences is not as indulgent as might be assumed (if one heeds traditional academic directives) because it provides a way to unravel lived experience with greater insight, that is, if it is conducted with 'honesty' and not a statement at the start to that effect. Here, honesty is seen in terms of an openness to one's own existing and potential flaws. Without meaning to transform the box step (used during some of the training manoeuvres in this research) into a soapbox, we do run the risk of teetering on the edge of what could be described as a fabricated construction of pseudo-academic expertise—one where academic practice has sought to emulate the 'expertise' offered by the self-proclaimed celebrity expert, one who, through their own self-declaration, is complicit in making a distinction between a world of 'celebrity' and the everyday 'ordinary' person. Sociologists (and academics in general) are not celebrities and nor should they attempt to emulate this vacuous construction which dominates contemporary western culture. If there is any value in making distinctions, these should be made in the form of distinguishing between what is considered research practice that maintains integrity and the superficiality of current, celebrity-obsessed, popular culture.

Experience of physical activity

As I mentioned in the introduction, sport has played a significant part in my life. Consequently, remaining mindful of my orientation towards physical activity is something that I have attempted to reflect upon and assess constantly throughout the decision-making processes that are continually being encountered. However, an important aspect of mindfulness about my own orientation to sport is the recognition that it is not necessarily always going to be the same as other men (or women) who 'love' sport. Continuing to take part in sport has often meant compromising and, in some cases, being complicit with the inequalities that I want to contest. This could be seen in the example that I gave in Chapter 7 relating to playing a tennis match with another man, whom I thought would harbour the same political convictions because the game was being played within the context of a gay tennis club. That I can 'do' sport has caused conflict, in that, on the one hand, it reinforces many forms of discrimination, but, on the other, it allows opportunities for me to 'fit in' and not draw unwanted attention to myself. Although I do not want to consciously promote discriminatory practices, being relatively 'good at sport' has meant that I have been able to participate without difficulty. As much as it caused internal turmoil, keeping my head down and not being outwardly gay in the stereotypical sense (precisely because this stereotype is associated with a non-sporting body) meant that life was relatively easy compared with the lives of many other gay men and women and, as such, I was able to continue to play sport. These dilemmas shaped the initial questions for my research into sporting masculinities, and subsequent research confirmed aspects of my own complicity, as well as that of the other gay men in the research who could perform 'expected' sporting masculinity (Wellard 2009). Consequently, it became apparent that the more I continued to take part in sport the greater the possibility that I might conform to the exclusionary practices that I was critical of in my academic writing. Connell (1995) describes the way that men can be complicit with hegemonic forms of masculinity although not necessarily expressing these in obviously aggressive or discriminatory forms. Therefore, it is important to recognise that my continued participation in sport means that I do conform (whether subtly or obviously, consciously or unconsciously) to a masculine agenda.

During the research that I conducted with men who played sport, it became clear that my own sexuality had not presented a barrier to my continued participation, unlike many of the other men whom I interviewed. Similarly, in my research relating to CrossFit, sexuality was not a barrier to participation either. It was apparent that my ability to 'do' sport has been a greater factor in my acceptance within sport and much of this relates to my outward bodily performances. To an extent, it could be claimed that during this research sexuality was put on the back burner because I had not considered it to be problematic. However, although sexuality was less evident on my research radar, age was much more apparent. Awareness of the ways in which age was a factor clearly affected the way that I continued with the research. Indeed, age dominated so many aspects of my experiences during the whole period. This included the physiological ways in which my body was able to cope with activities clearly aimed at a younger body. Even though the events in the Masters competitions had slightly reduced RX levels, the training programmes and expectations for performance were based on a model aimed at a 25-year-old body. The physical demands and expectations also played at the emotional level, particularly in terms of the subtle and not so subtle messages that appeared to present the older athlete as a separate entity.

It's still fun!

Although there is nothing new in the claim that participation in sport or physical activity is both subjective and complex, there remains a tendency, especially within popular culture, to ignore complexity in favour of simple or trite binaries (such as fit or unfit, healthy or obese, young or old, sporty or unsporty). Such generalisations impel the individual to form an allegiance with one or the other, and in doing so construct a sense of identification or dis-identification with the activity.

Nevertheless, despite awareness of the various barriers to participation and my academic sensibilities, I still enjoy sport and physical activity and make attempts to seek out ways to continue to do so. This 'will to sport' aspect was a main factor in my decision to undertake this research. I wanted to explore some of the ideas developed in *Sport, Fun and Enjoyment* (Wellard 2013), but in a more qualitative (personal) way. Although it is the case that many people want to take part in sports and physical activity, they do so for a variety of reasons. Health is not necessarily the main one, but rather working out what I can and cannot do, what I do and do not enjoy, just like everyone else, has been a central aspect in my continued relationship with it. Consequently, focusing on my own experiences assisted with my attempts to understand the processes through which an individual is constantly adapting, negotiating, compromising, enduring and tolerating—and, most importantly, enjoying an activity because, like me, they regard the experience to be worth it. Fun and enjoyment in this sense are not just a physical thrill or a means to maintain health—but also a mechanism to maintain an identity and a feeling of self-worth. Maybe, more tellingly, these activities offer a reminder of being alive. In the introduction, I mentioned the feelings of terror and excitement as a child diving into huge waves. These feelings are replicated when I hang upside down on a bar or attempt to hoist a ridiculously heavy weight (for me) over my head. Taken in this way, my research has not been about my own subjective experience, but rather an indication of not only the multiple ways in which a physical activity might be experienced, but also a hint of resistance to the restrictions on embodied experiences being placed on adults (and children).

Whose body is it anyway?

At face value, this book could be considered a subjective, personal account of *MY* body. Although this is the case to a certain extent, it is much more about the process of reflecting upon, accounting for and describing *A* body. Consequently, in giving over my body for the purposes of exploring an embodied experience, I am offering it as a focus of attention (or a subject) not only for my own scrutiny but also for others to scrutinise as they wish.

Seen from this perspective, my body is never my own, just like in everyday social interaction we are constantly presenting our bodies to others. Discourses of knowledge that operate around us conspire to make every aspect of our lives subject to some form of external gaze that dictates our everyday being. My body acts as a correspondent with my own perception of identity much as it does for others in the way that they are able to make sense of it. As post-structural accounts tell us, these identities are fluid and constantly changing, but not necessarily in a self-determined fashion. There are aspects of our identities that can be changed at will, but it is not always the case that an individually perceived transformation will be interpreted by others in the same way. Take the example of my beard. It may signal to me that I am making an outward gesture to others of a CrossFit identity. However, that presumes others will have a knowledge of what constitutes a CrossFit identity in the first place. It might just as easily represent a sign of old age or a general fashion statement. The point here is that, regardless of whether or not an identity can change, or what identity is being presented, it is, nevertheless, part of a performance. And, as such, the very fact that an identity warrants a performance of some kind—for others—means that a body is never going to belong to only the self.

The initial question 'whose body is it anyway?' seen in this light is counterproductive, because it positions control in terms of possession and ultimately promotes discussion about who has more control— whether this be the individual, other individuals, society in general or dominant groups. Although Foucault's concept of arbitrary systems of control that operate all the time provides a sophisticated and convincing theory to explain power, maybe we need to look beyond the limits of control.

What became clear during this research (and was an aspect of my previous research into fun and enjoyment) was the notion that intense engagement in physical activity on some occasions offered an 'escape' from everyday existence or a way to lose oneself. Here, I am once again reminded of Sartre's (1956) explanation that freedom is aligned with responsibility. Freedom in this interpretation is much more about the solitary individual, free to do as they choose, but this solipsistic existence is countered by the fact of being in a world of others, which ultimately demands a level of duty or responsibility to others. Seen in this light, freedom can be considered as an escape from responsibility and control. Consequently, the notion of transcendence that may occur in activities where one can 'lose oneself', such as an intense physical workout experienced in CrossFit, or other pursuits such as music and dance where one might get into a 'zone' (Jordan et al. 2017), offers a way of thinking about power as possibly less all encompassing.

Thus, the glimpses of 'freedom' that I experienced 'doing' CrossFit', as well as other sports (Wellard 2013), whether fleeting or temporary, are indications of a form of transcendence. These moments of being in a zone or being completely engulfed in a physical activity—where the rest of the world is shut out—might provide an insight into freedom in its purest form. In these moments of freedom, I do not need to care 'whose body it is anyway'.

REFERENCES

Ahmed, S. (2010) *The Promise of Happiness*. Durham, NC: Duke University Press.

Alcock, P. (2006) *Understanding Poverty*. Basingstoke, UK: Palgrave Macmillan.

Allen-Collinson, J. & Owton, H. (2014) Intense embodiment: Senses of heat in women's running and boxing. *Body and Society*, 1–24.

Allen-Collinson, J. & Owton, H. (2015) Intense embodiment: Senses of heat in women's running and boxing. *Body and Society*, **21**(2), 245–268.

Andrews, D.L. (1993) Desperately seeking Michel: Foucault's genealogy, the body, and critical sport sociology. *Sociology of Sport Journal*, **10**(2), 148–167.

Atkinson, M. (2010) Fell running in post-sport territories. *Qualitative Research in Sport and Exercise*, **2**(2), 109–132.

Atkinson, M. (2015) The loneliness of the fell runner. In: Wellard, I. (ed.), *Researching Embodied Sport: Exploring movement cultures*. London: Routledge.

Bailey, R. (2005) Physical education, sport and social inclusion. *Educational Review*, **57**(1), 71–90.

Bailey, R., Armour, K., Kirk, D., Jess, M., Pickup, I. & Sandford. R. (2009) The educational benefits claimed for physical education and school sport: An academic review. *Research Papers in Education*, **24**(1), 1–27.

Baker, J., Horton, S. & Weir, P. (2010) *The Masters Athlete*. London: Routledge.

Ball, S. (2004) Performativities and fabrications in the education economy: Towards the performative society. In: Ball, S. (ed.), *The RoutledgeFalmer Reader in Sociology of Education*. London: RoutledgeFalmer.

Barthes, R. (1977) *Image–Music–Text*. London: Fontana.

Bennett, T. (2006) Intellectuals, culture, policy: The technical, the practical, and the critical. *Cultural Analysis*, **5**, 1–5.

Bourdieu, P. (1984) *Distinction: A social critique of the judgment of taste*. Cambridge, MA: Harvard University Press.

Bourdieu, P. (1986) *Distinction*. London: Routledge.

Bourdieu, P. (1990) *The Logic of Practice*. Cambridge: Polity Press.

Bourdieu, P. & Wacquant, L. (1992) *An Invitation to Reflexive Sociology.* Cambridge: Polity Press.

Bourke, J. (2014) *The Story of Pain: From prayer to painkillers.* Oxford: Oxford University Press.

Brighton, J. (2014) Narratives of spinal cord injury and the sporting body: An ethnographic study. Unpublished PhD, Leeds Beckett University.

Butler, J. (1990) *Gender Trouble.* New York: Routledge.

Butler, J. (1993) *Bodies that Matter.* New York: Routledge.

Butler, J. (1997) *Excitable Speech.* New York: Routledge.

Carmichael, K. (1988) The creative use of pain in society. In: Teddington, R. (ed.), *Towards a Whole Society.* London: Fellowship Press.

Chaline, E. (2015) *The Temple of Perfection: A history of the gym.* London: Reaktion Books.

Clark, S. (2013) Running into trouble: Constructions of danger and risk in girls' access to outdoor space and physical activity. *Sport, Education and Society,* 20(8), 1012–1028.

Csikszentmihalyi, M. (1990) *Flow: The psychology of optimal experience.* New York: Harper Collins.

Connell, R.W. (1995) *Masculinities.* Cambridge: Polity Press.

Connell, R.W. (2005) *Masculinities,* 2nd edn. Cambridge: Polity Press.

Connell, R.W. (2007) *Southern Theory.* Cambridge: Polity.

Dawson, M. (2017) CrossFit: Fitness cult or reinventive institution? *International Review for the Sociology of Sport,* 52(3), 361–379.

de Beauvoir, S. (1972) *The Second Sex.* Harmondsworth: Penguin.

Delamont, S. (2005) No place for women among them? Reflections on the axé of fieldwork. *Sport, Education and Society,* 10(3), 305–320.

Department for Children, Schools and Families (2007) *The Children's Plan: Building brighter futures.* London: DCFS.

Department for Education and Skills (2004) *Every Child Matters: Change for children.* London: DfES.

Dolan, P. & Metcalfe, R. (2012) Measuring subjective wellbeing: Recommendations on measures for use by national governments. *Journal of Social Policy,* 41(2), 409–427.

Dornan, P. & Veit-Wilson, J. (2004) *Poverty: The facts.* London: Child Poverty Action Group.

Ellis, C. & Bochner, A.P. (2000) Autoethnography, personal narrative, reflexivity. In: Denzin, N.K. & Lincoln, Y.S. (eds), *Handbook of Qualitative Research,* 2nd edn. Thousand Oaks, CA: Sage, pp. 733–768.

Ereaut, G. & Whiting, R. (2008) What do we mean by 'wellbeing'? And why might it matter? DCSF Research Report No DCSF-RW073.

Evans, J. (2004) Making a difference? Education and 'ability' in physical education. *European Physical Review,* 10(1), 95–108.

Evans, J., Davies, B. & Wright, J. (2004) *Body Knowledge and Control.* London: Routledge.

Evers, C. (2015) Researching Action Sport with a GoPro™ Camera: An embodied and emotional mobile video tale of the sea, masculinity, and men-who-surf. In: Wellard, I. (ed.), *Researching Embodied Sport: Exploring movement cultures.* London: Routledge.

Featherstone, M. (1991) *The Body: Social process and cultural theory.* London: Sage.

Featherstone, M. (2010) Body, image and affect in consumer culture. *Body & Society*, 16(1), 193–221.

Firestone, S. (1979) *The Dialectic of Sex: The case for feminist revolution.* London: The Women's Press.

Foucault, M. (1978) *The History of Sexuality: An introduction.* Volume I. New York: Random House.

Foucault, M. (1979) *Discipline and Punish: The birth of the clinic.* London: Penguin Books.

Foucault, M. (1980) Truth and power. In: Gordon, C. (ed.), *Power/Knowledge: Selected interviews and other writings 1972–1977.* New York: Pantheon.

Foucault, M. (1985) *The Archaeology of Knowledge.* London: Tavistock Publications.

Frank, A. (1990) Bringing bodies back in: A decade review. *Theory, Culture and Society*, 7, 131–162.

Frank, A. (1991) For a sociology of the body: An analytical review. In: Featherstone, M., Hepworth, M. & Turner, B. (eds), *The Body: Social process and cultural theory.* London: Sage.

Furedi, F. (2008) *Paranoid Parenting.* London: Continuum Press.

Fussell, S. (1992) *Muscle.* London: Abacus.

Gard, M. (2006) Neither flower child nor artiste be: Aesthetics, ability and physical education. *Sport, Education and Society*, 11(3), 231–241.

Gard, M. (2011) A meditation in which consideration is given to the past and future engagement of social science generally and critical physical education and sports scholarship in particular with various scientific debates, including the so-called 'obesity epidemic' and contemporary manifestations of biological determinism. *Sport, Education and Society*, 16(3), 399–412.

Gard, M. & Wright, J. (2005) *The Obesity Epidemic: Science, morality and ideology.* London: Routledge.

Graham, G. (1995) Physical education through students' eyes and in students' voices: implications for teachers and researchers. *Journal of Teaching in Physical Education*, 14(4), 478–482.

Habermas, J. (1989) *The Structural Transformation of the Public Sphere. An Inquiry into a Category of Bourgeois Society.* Cambridge: Polity Press.

Hammersley, M. & Atkinson, P. (1995) *Ethnography, Principles in Practice.* London: Tavistock Publications.

Hargreaves, J. (1986) *Sport, Power and Culture.* London: Polity.

Hargreaves, J.A. (1994) *Sporting Females.* London: Routledge.

Heller, T., McCubbin, J.A., Drum, C. & Peterson, J. (2011) Physical activity and nutrition health promotion interventions: what is working for people with intellectual disabilities? *Intellectual and Developmental Disabilities*, 49(1), 26–36.

Howarth, D. (2013) *Poststructuralism and After: Structure, subjectivity and power.* Basingstoke: Palgrave Macmillan.

Humberstone, B. (2010) *Third Age and Leisure Research: Principles and practice.* LSA Publication No. 108. Eastbourne: Leisure Studies Association.

Hunter, I. (1994) *Rethinking the School. Subjectivity, Bureaucracy, Criticism.* Sydney: Allen & Unwin.

Jenkins, R. (1992) *Pierre Bourdieu.* London: Routledge.

Jordan, T., Woodward, K. & McClure, B. (2017) *Culture, Identity and Intense Performativity: Being in the zone.* London: Routledge.

Kafka, F. (2007) *Metamorphosis*. London: Penguin Modern Classics.

Kentel, J.A. & Dobson T.M. (2007) Beyond myopic visions of education: Revisiting movement literacy. *Physical Education and Sport Pedagogy*, 12(2), 145–162.

Kilgour, L., Matthews, N., Christian, P. & Shire, J. (2013) Health literacy in schools: Prioritising health and well-being issues through the curriculum. *Sport, Education and Society*, 20(4), 485–500.

Kirk, D. (1992) *Defining Physical Education: The social construction of a school subject in postwar Britain*. London: Falmer.

Knowles, Z. & Gilbourne, D. (2010) Aspiration, inspiration and illustration: Initiating debate on reflective practice writing. *The Sport Psychologist*, 24, 504–520.

Lester, S. & Russell, W. (2008) *Play for a Change: Play, policy and practice—a review of contemporary perspectives*. London: National Children's Bureau.

Low, J. & Malacrida, J. (2008) *Sociology of the body: A reader*. Oxford: Oxford University Press.

Markula, P. (2003) The technologies of the self: Sport, feminism, and Foucault. *Sociology of Sport Journal*, 20, 87–107.

Markula, P. & Pringle, R. (2006) *Foucault, Sport and Exercise: Power, knowledge and transforming the self*. London: Routledge.

Melzack, R. & Torgerson, W.S. (1971) On the language of pain. *Anesthesiology*, 34, 50–59.

Miller, J. (1994) *The Passion of Michel Foucault*. London: Flamingo.

Murphy, T.J. (2012) *Inside the Box: How CrossFit shredded the rules, stripped down the gym and rebuilt my body*. Boulder, CO: Velopress.

Nietzsche, F. (1969) On the genealogy of morals. In: *On the Genealogy of Morals and Ecce Homo* (transl. W. Kaufmannn & R.J. Hollingdale). New York: Vintage.

Nyaradi, A., Jianghong, L., Hickling, S., Foster, J. & Oddy, W.H. (2013) The role of nutrition in children's neurocognitive development, from pregnancy through childhood. *Frontiers in Human Neuroscience*, 7, 97.

Owen, G. (2006) Emotions and identities. In: Sport: Gay pride and shame in competitive rowing. Unpublished PhD, London South Bank University.

Phipps, A. (2014) *The Politics of the Body: Gender in a neoliberal and neoconservative age*. Cambridge: Polity Press.

Pickard, A. (2007) Girls, bodies and pain: Negotiating the body in ballet. In: Wellard, I. (ed.), *Rethinking Gender and Youth Sport*. London: Routledge, pp. 36–50.

Pill, S. (2010) Sport literacy: It's not just about learning to play sport via 'textbook techniques'. *Journal of Student Wellbeing*, 4(2), 32–42.

Plummer, K. (2010) *Sociology: The basics*. London: Routledge.

Powell, S. & Wellard, I. (2008) *Policies and Play: The impact of national policies on children's opportunities for play*. London: Play England and the National Children's Bureau.

Pringle, R. & Markula, P. (2005) 'No Pain is Sane After All': A Foucauldian analysis of masculinities and men's experiences in rugby. *Sociology of Sport Journal*, 22, 472–497.

Pronger, B. (2002) *Body Fascism: Salvation in the technology of fitness*. Toronto: University of Toronto Press.

Rose, N. (1999) *Powers of Freedom: Reframing political thought*. Cambridge: Cambridge University Press.

Rose, N. (2007) *The Politics of Life Itself: Biomedicine, power, and subjectivity in the twenty-first century*. Princeton, NJ: Princeton University Press.

Sallis, J. & Owen, N. (1999) *Physical Activity and Behavioral Medicine*. Thousand Oaks, CA: Sage.

Sartre, J.-P. (1956) *Being and Nothingness: An essay on phenomenological ontology*. New York: Philosophical Library.

Segal, L. (1997) *Slow Motion: Changing masculinities, changing men*. London: Virago.

Shilling, C. (1993) *The Body and Social Theory*. London: Sage.

Shilling, C. (2008) *Changing Bodies: Habit, crisis and creativity*. London: Sage.

Smith Maguire, J. (2002) Michel Foucault: Sport, power, technologies and governmentality. In: Maguire, J.A. & Young, K. (eds), *Theory, Sport and Society*. Oxford: Elsevier Science Ltd, pp. 293–314.

Smith Maguire, J. (2008) The personal is professional. *International Journal of Cultural Studies*, 11(2), 211–229.

Sobchack, V. (2004) *Carnal Thoughts: Embodiment and moving image culture*. Berkeley, CA: University of California Press.

Sparkes, A.C. (1996) The fatal flaw: A narrative of the fragile body-self. *Qualitative Inquiry*, 2, 463–494.

Sparkes, A.C. (2002) *Telling Tales in Sport and Physical Activity: A qualitative journey*. Champaign, IL: Human Kinetics.

Sparkes, A.C. (2007) Embodiment, academics, and the audit culture: A story seeking consideration. *Qualitative Research*, 7(4), 521–550.

Sport England (2017) 'Active Lives Adult Survey, May 16/17 Report'. Available at: www.sportengland.org/media/12458/active-lives-adult-may-16-17-report.pdf.

Sport Wales (2010) 'A Vision for Sport in Wales'. Available at: http://sport.wales/media/506916/sport_wales_english_vision_doc_reprint_all_v3.pdf.

Stamford, B. (1987) No pain, no gain? *Physician and Sportmedicine*, 15, 244.

Stebbins, R.A. (2006) *Serious Leisure: A perspective of our time*. New Brunswick, NJ: Transaction Publishers.

Synnott, A. (1993) *The Body Social*. London: Routledge.

Taussig, G. (1991) Tactility and distraction. *Cultural Anthropology*, 6(2), 147–153.

Tennant, R., Hiller, L., Fishwick, R. et al. (2007) The Warwick-Edinburgh Mental Well-being Scale (WEMWBS): Development and UK validation. *Health and Quality of Life Outcomes*, 5, 63. Available from: www.hqlo.com/content/5/1/63.

Tolkien, J.R.R. (1992) *The Lord of the Rings*. London: Grafton.

Tomlinson, A. (1990) *Consumption, Identity & Style*. London: Routledge.

Urry, J. (1995) *Consuming Places*. London: Routledge.

Vernon, M. (2008) *Wellbeing*. Stocksfield: Acumen.

Wellard, I. (2002) Men, sport, body performance and the maintenance of 'exclusive masculinity'. *Leisure Studies*, 21, 235–247.

Wellard, I. (2006) Able bodies and sport participation: social constructions of physical ability. *Sport, Education and Society*, 11(2), 105–119.

Wellard, I. (2009) *Sport, Masculinities and the Body*. New York: Routledge.

Wellard, I. (2013) *Sport, Fun and Enjoyment: An embodied approach*. London: Routledge.

Whannel, G. (2006) The four minute mythology: Documenting drama on film and television. *Sport in History*, 26(2), 263–279.

Whannel, G. & Wellard, I. (1995) Sports stars and popular mythologies. *20:20*, 1.

Wheaton, B. (2004) *Understanding Lifestyle Sports: Consumption, Identity and Difference*. London: Routledge.

Whitehead, M. (2010) *Physical Literacy*. London: Routledge.

Woodward, K. (2015) Bodies in the zone. In: Wellard, I. (ed.), *Researching Embodied Sport: Exploring movement cultures*. London: Routledge.

Young, I.M. (1980) Throwing like a girl: A phenomenology of feminine body comportment motility and spatiality. *Human Studies*, 3(2), 137–156.

Youth Sport Trust (2013) *Primary School Physical Literacy Framework*. Available at: www.youthsporttrust.org/media/5174173/physical_literacy_framework.pdf.

INDEX